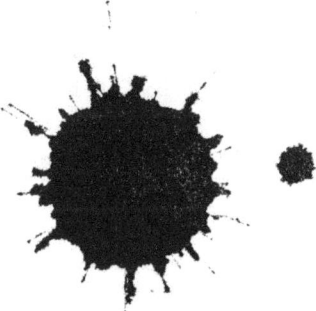

THROWING UP RAINBOWS

My Eating Disorder and Other Colorful Things

Z ZOCCOLANTE

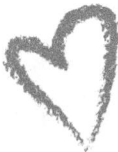

DREAM
BIG
BOOKS

Lyrics to "Fuel" by Ani Difranco, In Little Plastic Castle, Righteous Babe, 1998, compact disk. Used with permission. Frost, Robert. "A Servant to Servants" in North of Boston (New York: Henry Holt, 1917), p. 64. Used with permission.

Dream Big Books
PO BOX 1594
El Segundo, CA 90245
www.dreambigbooks.love
info@dreambigbooks.love

Library of Congress Control Number: 2018907586

ISBN: 978-1-7324536-0-9

Printed in the United States of America

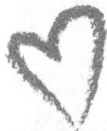

DREAM
BIG
BOOKS

This is for us all, who exposed our darkest fears.

For those who are still crawling, know you are not alone.

CONTENTS

INTRODUCTION

Every story has a villain. Every story has a hero. I am both.

My name is Christen but I go by Z. For eleven and a half years I devoted my whole being to my secret love affair with anorexia and bulimia. I felt that if people saw who I thought I was, all dirty, dark, and ugly on the inside, no one would like me.

When I was in the disorder, I believed there was a magic key that would grant me the happiness and freedom I longed for. For years, I kept volumes of secrets hidden in the pages of my journals, but I couldn't stop the behavior. Eating disorders gain power and thrive in secrecy. They keep you feeling worthless and hopeless. They make you hide from those who love you.

When I finally got over my shame to the degree that I could buy books on eating disorders, the stories left me with more questions than answers. It infuriated me when people alluded to just giving it to God. If God wanted it, why didn't He take it away when I lay sobbing on my carpet? Most books ended with the authors leaving the hospital and accepting they would live with the disease forever. The books ended where I thought they should begin. If I fought for my freedom, I wanted a version of happily ever after that included an element of finality.

I wanted to write the missing story of what happens during recovery and what comes after. My story begins at the hospital and traverses my therapy, family, and marriage during and after recovery. These pages provide a secret window into the twisting war of my eating disorder. They speak my heart's truth—all the raw, angry, and dark feelings. It's the story I would have wanted to hear.

If you are watching someone struggling with an eating disorder, my hope is that this book will give you insight and compassion to support those you love. If you are struggling with an eating disorder, may you find what you need in these pages to ignite a fiery spark towards your own recovery. I will not lie to you. There is a place of freedom, peace, joy and happiness. Please do whatever it takes to get there. Do whatever it takes to be free. Know that I support your journey with all my heart. Know that I love you. Know that God loves you. If you have picked up this book, it's your time. Freedom is calling your name.

No more secrets. No more pain. Live free. Live on.

With love,
Z :)

A NOTE ON CHARACTERS

All of the people in my story have contributed powerfully to my recovery. I hold each of them with admiration, love, and gratitude. No eating disorder is ever an isolated, solo tale. I have endeavored respectfully to protect people's identities and individual stories. Several requested that their names be omitted or changed.

For the privacy of hospital staff and patients, I have not mentioned the name of the institution. The names and physical descriptions of these hospital staff members have been altered: Jackie, Margaret, Rachel, the anger workshop facilitator, and the nutritionist/dietician. I've referred to all of the women patients as girls, despite varying ages. The patient names Julie, Ellie, and Sara are pseudonyms.

Other persons who requested pseudonyms or anonymity are my former roommate, Sebastian; my psychologist and neurofeedback specialist; my cognitive behavioral therapist, and my marriage and family therapist before entering the hospital. My places of work are also unnamed.

The following names have not been changed: my husband, Leon; my brother, Zack; Pastor Larry; my main clinical psychologist and eating disorder specialist, Liza; and my friends, Di and Mel.

Correctly identified in my story are Leon's father, grandmother, sister, uncle, and grandparents. Also willing to be included without obscuring their identities were a college friend, my brother's girlfriend, Di's mother and uncle, former clients, a man I met on vacation, my landlord, my yoga teacher, a boy and his mother encountered at a family gathering, and my mother and father.

PROLOGUE

I know my mind is sick because the words tell me so. They spill my disorder in the seclusion of the bathroom, where I rub cold water against my face to feel clean again. The girl in the mirror stares through me. I don't meet her eyes. I hate that she sees past my smile. She recites the words in the bowl of sadness, before it swirls down the drain.

*

Half a gallon of ice cream, chocolate cake frosted with pink speckled clouds, raw brownie batter, water, potato chips, three glazed doughnuts, pasta shells (the middles hard as stone) drowning in linguini, brown rice with mustard and ketchup and olive oil, five pieces of bread with jam and honey, two handfuls of red grapes, an empty heart, a pretty face.

The words recycle on my command, over my tongue, past my teeth, exploding in a whisper. The soft plunk of a rainbow into water, the familiar sound comfort makes. Cradling the porcelain, my hair falls down in little streaks of sunshine, the straw tips of paintbrushes having come undone. Last, the grapes bleed from my throat like wine and watery corpses the color of rose petals. The grapes, the first that went in my stomach, mark the beginning. I've rewound time. It's all out now. I can stop.

Elation fills me and quickly subsides. I pick my head up in shame; cradle it in hands of self-hatred. In a moment of lucidity, I attach to myself again, and for an instant, I get a glimpse, I see the reality that I could be so much more; that I'm wasting my life, and I don't know how to stop. What I could have been now, at age 24 . . . I could have been beautiful.

Today will not be the day I die. This makes me only slightly happy. If the grapes had a voice they would say, "you can stop now, you're in control again; relax your mind."

Downstairs, the last pint of ice cream melts. Clear glass bowls cover the countertop, clumps of color clinging to their insides. A twisty-tie, a half empty bag of bread, an uncovered container of jam, and the remnants of jars I must finish whole or waste. Everything salvageable gets put back in its place. Every dish is washed clean, the strange putting back of time. Everything else deserves a new plastic bag, the one I hold as I creep down the block to the perfect trashcan where my partner would never think to look. I must do all this between two hands on the clock. I must do all this in the whisper of the explosion. I must do all this in the silence between my partner and me. I must do all this because in less than fifteen minutes he'll plagiarize my counterfeit smile and wander through our kitchen, inspect our dish rack, and count the dishes.

*

When he walks through the door the word *skinny* lingers. Its frequency is specific. He's unaware how full the room is, the weight and space words carry.

I cannot unlearn this language of words. They whisper. They scream. They're a constant. They pound beneath my skin in frantic melody reaching for my heart, arching gnarled fingers, plucking across my ribs like symphony strings. Peace has become a word I recognize only when sounding out the letters.

My smile is a brilliant blue star. I am the pathetic failure collapsing with the guilt of being found out. He's holding a flat cardboard box. He sets it on the table. Beneath the cellophane is a huge chocolate chip cookie. The red letter icing spells out, "Happy Anniversary Peanut." He makes me promise that it'll last at least a week. He tries to trust me and treat me like a normal person.

When he goes to sleep I sneak downstairs. I eat other things so I don't break my promise about the cookie. A halo from the kitchen light reflects off the cellophane. I can trust myself with one bite. Then one more . . .

The words follow me up the stairs. The one who loves me is asleep in our bed. His eyelashes flicker, gold at the tips. My feet trace the carpet. I am a shadow. I am the wind. The sheets are cold under my palm. He shifts his arms around the pillow at his chest. My heart spikes. I am a deer. I am nothing.

I back away from the bed, across the carpet, through the open door, down the hallway to the bathroom. I shut myself in with the lights off. There's a sliver of white light at the bottom of the door. I twist the shower on hot and fold under the watery flames. Darkness surrounds me but I cannot escape the words.

You do not deserve him. You are weak. You are worthless. You lie. You always lie.

I put my fingers in my ears and press until it hurts, until there's silence. When I take my hands away from my face, hot raindrops slide down my skin. There's a blessed pause, an interlude where the alternate reality of my life plays before my eyes. I am with the one who loves me. We are laughing. My smile is honest. Happiness overwhelms me making it hard to breathe. And then . . . *Skinny.*

When I turn off the water the steam presses into my lungs. I leave a trail of wet footprint on the floor. Eyes closed, my finger slides along the mirror. I pretend I'm spelling the words in blood on a scroll that will bind me for all time.

I flick on the light. My pupils' retract. The letters are bleeding at the edges but the message is clear. I need help. I place the end of my finger between my teeth reviewing my work of art. I add one single dot, touching my finger to the mirror, after the words. The period makes all the difference. It's now a decision, complete at the end. I cannot do this on my own.

I need help.

PART ONE

1

THE WORDS THAT KEEP ME FROM SLEEPING

Having been married one year and two days exactly, Leon buys me a huge sixteen-inch chocolate chip cookie with icing that spells in red letters, "Happy Anniversary, Peanut."

"This should last you at least a week," he says, because he tries to trust me and treat me like a normal person.

"I know," I say, slightly annoyed. "I'll eat half tonight and save the other half till the last night of this week."

"That's not even funny," he says.

"I know. I know," I laugh.

"Promise me."

"I promise already."

He wants to have sex, but all I can think about is the cookie and how I hate him for making me promise, because I know the one thing in life I should be able to control, my eating, is the one thing I can never get right. This body that fails me is a constant torture. My ass grows fat and rippled. I lie. I'm a bad person. I try so hard.

"Why does it matter?" he says. "You're not fat at all. You've got a beautiful body."

"You're biased because you want sex," I say.

"Goodnight," he says.

"Whatever," I say.

"I just don't want to lose you when you're thirty or forty. What happens when you die and I'm left all alone?"

"Then you can find someone else to be with who's not messed up like me, and you can have sex all day long."

"I don't want someone else. I want you."

"Goodnight," I say.

"Whatever," he says.

What's wrong with me? He's so good to me, and I'm a big fat liar. If I love him, shouldn't I be able to stop? If I love him enough, why doesn't this fact stop me?

He's already sleeping as I inch on my side of the bed as far away physically as I can push from the heat of his body. His oval face presses into the pillow as I stare at the arch of his eyebrow, his lashes that lighten from brown to blond at the tips. I used to adore the freckle on his cheek. It reminded me of a star and the constellations we watched while we were dating, when everything was electric and happy. I follow the curve of his slender frame down his long runner's leg and watch his toes twitch and curl inwards on themselves like a baby monkey's hand.

It must be exhausting for him to watch me killing myself. I try not to think about it. I try to sleep, but sleep is a tease because my first thought upon awaking is *fuck,* and a flood of despair pools in. When I wake from my peaceful dreams, I know what I've become.

As usual, our comforter has shifted towards his side of the bed, underneath the dead weight of his leg, and I can't pull it free. This fact enrages me now, because it gets so cold here in California with its pathetic little excuses for palm trees that look like pineapples with stilts up their butts. Now, in the cold, I notice all the white space along our walls, the lack of furniture, the hollow places love should fill. We don't have enough of anything to fill the emptiness. It's the biggest place I've ever lived in, coming from a small apartment in Hawai'i that housed all four people in my family and overflowed with stuff.

I hate words because I love them, because they keep me from sleeping, because they keep me staring at the empty shell-white walls of our home, hearing over and over his words that say I lack passion. Words speak of my other problems, like eating ice cream.

I know it's not funny how I creep downstairs. I know it's not funny how I hide the cookie box in the oven, hoping out of sight really does mean out of mind. I know it's not funny, the little deals I make with myself to give me permission to gorge on other foods, so I don't break my promise about the cookie. It's also not funny when I have a bowl of ice cream and think I can trust myself with a small section of my anniversary present, and then just one more...

Stop you can't do this. You promised, I say.

I lied, I say.

But you promised, I say.

Fine, I say.

After eating most of the box of ice cream, I exorcise its milky brown puddles, which begin to curdle before falling down the garbage disposal I've clogged two times. My mind rewinds past all the people I've disappointed and drops me in a field under the sun. I'm eight years old teetering at the top of the hill as my dad gives me a gentle push. I ride a blue Smurf tricycle as it zooms over the grass, its little wheels spinning frantically, the wind pulling my exhilarated screeches through the air. Eyes wide, I am laughing; my dad is laughing, too, running down the hill. The sensation of forgotten freedom overwhelms me like stones in my belly as I begin to cry, holding it in so my throat swells.

I turn on the water and wash it down: the ice cream, the blue Smurf tricycle, the people I've disappointed. They fall over the edge straight down into the pipes. I hate words because they form images that I cannot shake: blue Smurf, freedom. But the words I hate tonight are Leon's.

An hour ago, he took my hand and renewed his vows, the cookie as witness. I let my hand drop in silence, which was all I could do to keep myself from wailing.

I wish I could crawl through the spirals of time and live again in those memories of freedom, when I was pure and good. When I loved life and lived free. When I didn't lie or hurt people or myself. When I was happy. Before the sorrow and the grief and whatever else grew inside me, blurring and smearing the beautiful girl that I was.

I was about fifteen when I fell into the hole. Two years later, by my junior year of high school, I'd already taught myself how to throw up by turning my stomach. I had transitioned from anorexia to bulimia in secret; on the outside people thought I was recovering because I ate. My parents were the only ones who knew my secret. After school, when my mom picked me up, we went together around the block to Baskin Robbins, where we had enjoyed many an afterschool conversation over ice cream. Angst filled me. The shop had no bathroom, and I would have to hold it until I got home. As we sat at the table, her face was hopeful with the anticipation of spending time with me, the naiveté that came from thinking she could fix something by willing it to be different and then pretending it was. I could almost hear the crack in my heart her voice made.

She couldn't bring herself to say, "Please don't throw this up," so what she said was, "How was your day at school?"

I tried hard to put on a pretty face, not to be moody and short on the way home, not to be mean and hurtful with my indifference.

Years later, but still not recovered, I had to look away as she wrestled with the fear that it was her fault I had become anorexic.

"Was it anything I did?" She wanted me to tell her it wasn't. She wanted me to tell her it was OK, to assuage her guilt. I didn't comply.

"Interesting," was all I said, even though it wasn't her fault. There is no fault.

All the many afternoons we got ice cream, all the money she spent, all the rides in the car, all the simple questions that masked darker concerns, all the time and the sacrifice and the love she tried to give me in ice cream, and I could not remember one conversation we'd had. It was like she wasn't even there.

2

SPIRAL

Christen—

I love you, and I want you to get better. I know you know you have a problem, but I don't think you know the severity. I know it hasn't stopped. I think you are in a form of denial. You cannot fight your body without consequences. I know it's not going to be fixed by some symbolic word telling you to stop, because it is not that easy. Time will not heal this. You need to seek help. It can be kept quiet, no one in the family needs to know, and doctors can help. I am here for you. Let's do this. Let's fix it.

—Leon

I feel like I'm suffocating as I sit outside the coffee shop where I work part-time while I finish esthetics school. The dim light of the afternoon sun tries to break through the smoky dust-colored cotton ball clouds. Outside, I find the one table hidden in the corner under an awning of vines. My eyes burn with anger and not enough sleep. I am unraveling like a dirty ball of yarn.

People know. When I blink I still abhor myself because I'm always so careful, and the other night at the party, I was not.

Leon and I had arrived in the late afternoon. We'd made our way to the open air of his uncle's lanai. A seal was swimming out towards the horizon, popping up its slick black head through the gray water.

At first, I'd munched on blueberries, cherries, and strawberries—all the fruit we couldn't afford to buy for ourselves. As more people arrived, the table had filled with appetizers, Brie and crackers, stuffed olives, little quiche tarts, breads, and creamy dips. I had filled my small plate sparingly with a few olives, a piece of bread, and a little dip, but then the younger guests had arrived and I had needed to make conversation with people I didn't know well, which made me anxious and insecure. I'd laughed and smiled like everything was normal, as I went back for heavier foods that I didn't normally eat, the Brie, the quiche tarts. When I swallowed the first tart I'd known the spiral had begun.

I'd been aware of the rising anxiety—of having to pretend that everything was fine, that I was enjoying the party the same way as everyone else—all the while being focused on only one thing: when I could grab another bite. The more anxious I'd become, the more I'd wanted people to go away, so I could devour all the food and throw it all up.

Methodically I'd taken bite after small bite, becoming more detached until the party was white noise and my head became the room. Bits and pieces of conversations filtered in, something about reviving someone whose heart had stopped. Wildly interesting, but there had been no time to ask questions, because conversation would have interrupted my controlled bites. A white tablecloth, the blood red of the cherries, the Christmas ornaments. I'd pretended to be interested in all of them so I could avoid conversation. Sneaking off to both bathrooms, checking the locks to make sure they were secure, the flush of the toilets, my face in the mirror as I'd pep-talked myself into going back out and avoiding the food.

Dinner and dessert were served as the sky turned from gray to black, and the fireworks started. Distraction and darkness provided cover, so I could eat more dessert without being obvious. Finally we'd moved inside to open presents. My hand held red and green M&Ms. I'd popped them into my mouth, but by that time I was the only one still eating. The cycle had resumed in full momentum. Had I been alone, I would have sat and eaten all the M&Ms, all the desserts, and all the appetizers, shoving them into my mouth like a feral animal that hadn't eaten in weeks.

As Leon and I drove home that night, I was exhausted from pretending. I had stared out the window and watched the ocean scroll by, the anxiety racing, still wanting more. I'd hated myself, but silently I'd congratulated myself for having made it through another party without letting on that I had this disorder. I thought I'd held my appearance together quite well. I had smiled and laughed at all the appropriate times. I'd drunk lots of water to have an excuse to use the restroom. But a day or two after the party, when I got home from work, Leon had sat me down on our green velvet couch. My heart had started to drum. What could he have found— specks in the toilet, missing food, a clogged sink, my secret trashcan?

He'd taken a breath. His soft lips had said his uncle had called to say people at the party expressed concern about my excessive trips to the bathroom. Every organ in me had tightened and numbed.

People know. People know. People know, my mind shouted as I'd flipped through my memories of the party. *No. No. No.*

Leon had spent the morning researching my disorder and typing out exactly how I would die if I didn't stop. He'd handed me a letter pleading with me to get help. When he'd said "sudden death," his words had floated like oil on water, sitting on the surface, heavy and thick, but not touching me.

A thorny vine had worked its way from my stomach to my throat, but I would not cry in front of him, so I'd pretended to ignore him. I had sat perfectly, painfully still as my mind flooded and drowned. *His uncle should mind his own fucking business.* My hatred had been visceral, like a razor blade slicing a vein. I had focused on my rage until everything else numbed out, until the hatred was all I could taste.

Leon's green eyes had bored into the side of my face, pleading. Exhausted, he'd closed them and dropped his head, brown curls escaping through the spaces between his fingers. I'd picked one point on the table and stared at it like my life depended on it. Maybe if I'd waited long enough I could have made the whole moment disappear. The silence had gone on until he gave up waiting for me to respond and trudged upstairs, leaving the letter on the table. I'd considered tearing it to shreds, but deeper down a sorrow had imploded. I couldn't be there but I couldn't go anywhere else.

Instead, I'd stepped out to our car in the garage, a little coffin inside a bigger coffin. I'd locked myself in and turned the stereo up until I felt the vibration in my bones, and at just the right moment, I'd screamed, electrifying every particle of air around me. In the violence of my scream, I was everything I'd ever wanted to be and gave up trying to become.

*

At the coffee shop, my break is over. Leon and I haven't spoken since the confrontation two nights earlier. Rain begins to fall from gray clouds that hover. I feel so defeated, all my insecurities split open. I am someone who needs help, and I am embarrassed that Leon had to get a stupid phone call from his nosy uncle. What upsets me most is that I'm such a failure. I'm upset that I can't be his perfect person. I'm ashamed that he married me.

My silver car sits lonely in the parking lot, repelling raindrops like a duck's feathers. I have a feeling he said he wanted the car tonight, but I can't bring myself to drive home or to call him and ask. Pathetic little me—fake, deteriorated inside, tragically flawed, insecure, stupid. *People know.*

My break is over. As I put my apron back on and walk behind the counter, my pretend smile is part of my costume. The espresso machine clicks as I pull the lever back. A small clump of dirt-like coffee grounds falls down into the metal circle. I smash and turn it like a poi pounder. Pushing the circle up into its fitting, I turn my wrist hard to the right locking it in place. The buttons remind me of the slightly puffy dials on massage chairs. When I push them, the machine comes to life, taking in a breath as the earthy scent expands and espresso foams into little shot glasses. I look out the windows. My car is gone, but Leon's motorcycle holds the spot. Later, I look again. My car is back, and Leon's bike is gone.

The espresso machine lets out its exhausted last breath, and the drizzle on the windows makes my silver car blur into a gray sky. *He didn't come in to see me. I've gone too far. He doesn't want me anymore.* Staring between the rain droplets on the window, I picture my life without him, never again knowing the amazing lightness of hearing him talk to our cat, his baby voice floating up the stairs surrounding my heart, happiness overtaking me just for an instant. Or the way he hugs me goodbye before I leave for work early in the morning, sleepy-eyed, hair in frazzles, rambling incoherent things, delirious from dreaming. Who would I be without those simple things and the lightness they bring?

Light flows through any opening, even if it's only the size of a pinprick. I am the one fully responsible if he wants out of the marriage.

But I can change, I say.

No you can't, I say.

You lie, I say.

You always lie, I say.

That's who you are, I say. *A Big Fat Liar.*

If I could breathe in the rain, I would inhale it in gulps and flood my lungs, keeping focused through the panic, doing it for him, because he would be better off without me.

When my shift at the coffee shop ends, I walk unhurried towards my car, the raindrops cold and beading like tiny pearls on my eyelashes. On the front seat, instead of emptiness there is something—the piece of paper with our marriage promises and some handpicked flowers.

At twenty-four, my mom was picking little yellow daisies for my dad and finding him in the college cafeteria by the sound of his guitar. They were just starting their love story.

At twenty-four, I am sitting in my car in the rain with a reminder of the marriage promises I've broken and some handpicked flowers. It feels like the solidifying of an ending, tangible proof that I am a failure as a wife and person. When I realize he's going to fight for us, the anger seeps back in, but why am I mad? He knows me, and I hate people who know. I hate that I let someone get close enough to see all my dirty secrets. Why can't people see just the fake me—all smiles and long blonde hair and skin a nice brown from living in Hawai'i? Fake me is always enchanting, not broken or wounded.

Leon fell in love with the beautiful side of me and now he's seeing the ugliness. I push people away as soon as they get close, keep them at a distance far enough that they never really know. Sometimes I push away violently, most times with nothing more than a shrug. The anger seeps in because I can't be normal, because I can't look him in the face and have it be the same. Because now I know how he'll see me, all shattered inside. He'll watch me, and each time I look at him, I'll see the part of me I hate reflected back.

*

When I arrive home, my mind is spinning, but my mouth won't form any of the words. It's easier not to admit out loud that I'm a pathetic waste. Instead of going upstairs where he is, I plop down on the green velvet couch and turn on the TV. After an hour, he trudges down the stairs and stands there staring at me as I stare at the TV.

"How long are you going to ignore me?"

I stay silent.

"I don't feel I deserve this."

I look at him blankly and turn back to the TV. *Of course you don't. I should have known better than to get married and ruin two lives.*

He walks away.

3

THE LINE I'D ALWAYS WANTED TO CROSS

My hair is jet black. The blonde hair I had this morning now matches my black eyebrows, making my eyes pull the color blue out of the hazel. Somehow I always knew I'd be doing this. Painting my eyelids like a cat, tracing tar around my eyes, smoothing a deep purple blood color against my lips. Painting myself the colors I feel inside, my teeth blinding white against my lips.

I have lived for eleven years with a voice in my head—a woman who has been trying to kill me. Naming her made her feel like an outside entity, somehow not part of the good person who was still me.

She first came to me when I was fifteen. She was blonde, dressed like a fairy, and so pretty. She promised me that I could be all I ever wanted if I was just a little thinner. She didn't tell me her name then, but she adopted mine, and my voice, and she hollowed me out into a shell perfectly fit for her.

At first I didn't complain; I felt special. But she didn't let me eat what I wanted, and I had to go on longer and longer runs, and I wasn't happy anymore. Then Lillie came to me. She was my savior, or so I thought. She was the one who seduced me into what I thought was the great discovery of spitting out food so that I could taste forbidden things again, like dessert. However spitting is frowned upon when others are present, so Lillie gave me the brilliant idea that I could throw up only dessert.

"Just stick your fingers down your throat, touch the little hangy ball, and gag

it all up." Lillie protected me from the teasing at school, when I couldn't stand up for myself. She was angry and bitter and powerful, and I loved her.

When Lillie came to me the first time she was blonde and dressed like a fairy, and she had borrowed my name. But when the disguise no longer worked, she showed herself in the moonlight—black hair, black dress, black eyes, purple lips. Powerful, seductive, magic, and she chose me to be her friend. I believed she could help me become powerful, that I could eat and still have everything I wanted. She made me believe it was possible. And then she turned on me.

Now I am Lillie. The black hair completes the image. It's how I'd always pictured her. Cutting my hair was taboo. It was one of those things I was conditioned not to do.

"Why do you want to do that?" my parents would ask. "Your hair is so pretty the way it is. Don't you think? Don't cut your hair. Don't dye your hair. Don't drink. Don't smoke. Don't ever have sex. Don't ever get a tattoo. Why do you always dress down? You could be so much prettier if you only . . . Don't you think it's better this way?"

It seems almost too simple, but my hair is a metaphor for two things: I no longer feel I have anything to lose, and I have reached a point with Lillie that her darkness is finally taking over. As I find myself trying so hard to be good, which means not throwing up, I also find myself binging in front of the TV with the urgency to stuff down all the food in the house and bring it back up. *Why? Why? Why?*

All the while, I try so hard to keep Lillie a secret, and to hold my marriage together. It hangs delicately like a spider's web with lots of vacant space, and I'm scared every tiny raindrop will cause its collapse. Lillie crawls like the black widow she is, bundles me tightly with the strands of her web and whispers to me incessantly until I break.

When I succeed and can filter out Lillie's voice for brief moments, I spend it planning romantic attempts at candlelit dinners, evenings of blindfold escapades, and massages with happy endings. I put on my most pretty mask, ignore the dialogue in my head, and pretend that I am normal. Sex is what I think I must provide to maintain the relationship I have, a begrudged offering that I give over to keep the peace. Life has become a long, exhausting string of loving Leon and hating me.

Sometimes when the TV is on, I lose huge gaps in time while I methodically shovel food down my throat, remembering Christmases when, as a kid, I listened to Christian Psalty tapes. I see rainy days when my mom would place a velvet curtain in the doorway of our room and give my brother and me puppet shows about a little silver unicorn with a purple horn who wanted to be a rock star. The little unicorn was a finger puppet, and he would jump out from his mom's pouch like a kangaroo joey and sing, "I wanna be a rock starrrrrrr!" His mom would always try to put him back in the pouch because he was interrupting her story, but out he would pop with the same line. And Zack and I would laugh and laugh. I try to shove these memories down with the food, but they keep haunting me with the happiness I no longer have. It's funny how certain things represent freedom and the possibility of my dreams coming true—a blue Smurf tricycle, a unicorn finger puppet with a purple horn.

When Lillie took over my life, I still had my dreams, and in them I was free. Now sleep, too, teases me because even in my dreams, I have the same addictions. During weeks when I can be good for a few days, my dreams are of buffet tables laden with all the desserts I could ever want. Sometimes when I resist, I wake up and think, *Damn it. I could have eaten it all and not paid the price.* Other times while dreaming, I do eat it all and throw it up, and I wake up feeling like the failure I've become.

Although Lillie is with me, my dreams haven't caught up with my married life, because in them I always start out single and only remember right at the end, usually propelled by my attraction to some random stranger, that I do in fact have a husband.

*

Christmas Day. This is a rotten Christmas. I found out how unhappy Leon is to be with me. As I place his gifts from Santa by the bed, he says he didn't get me anything. I just want to make him happy. I put on my blue sweatpants because I don't want jeans constricting my stomach, pressing against me reminding me how fat I am, making me hate myself. He hates the sweatpants, and he brings me a different shirt as I change. I ask for my pants back. I want to wear my blue sweater but know he'll disapprove, so I pick out a red Christmassy one. He looks me over when I emerge from the closet. "All of your clothes are hand-me-downs, aren't they?" he accuses. *It's brand new!* I want to shout and push him out the window, because he hurts my feelings.

At his grandparents' house we have a yummy dinner, but Leon isn't lovey with me anymore. On the drive home he doesn't answer me when I ask if he's happy to be with me, but I know he's not. After he's silent for a while, I ask him why he doesn't love me anymore, and he begins a long tangent about how he's reached the point where he's not happy with me. He's lost the passion, our sex life sucks, I never dress up, I can't clean. He throws in little things I can't do, like peeling a potato tonight. Since when did peeling a potato become a life skill, or a marriage qualification? I've never once heard a guy say, "Yeah, she's fantastic, but I'm going to have to break up with her. She just can't peel a potato."

On the flip side, he says that when I want to, I can be the most loving person. There's more, but I don't hear it. When I fade back into the conversation, he's telling me that if our sex doesn't get better, our marriage will fall apart. *So basically I suck as a wife.* But he does love me, he adds.

My throat burns and I can't swallow the hard knot lodged there as I struggle to silence myself so I don't start to cry. I feel awful and the thought comes again, *I wish I'd never gotten married.* Leon was attracted to me because I shined, but then he got bored when he realized I was only a penny.

He had asked me what I wanted for Christmas, and I'd told him a massage, but a free one from him. It's around 9:00 p.m., and I apprehensively ask him about it. He goes upstairs and brings down an envelope. "Here," he says, dropping it on the coffee table as he walks away. Even though he's drawn a little sketch of a peanut—his nickname for me—on the front, and the back reads, "I heart you," I can feel that it's cold. Against the pure white envelope I notice my fingernails, bitten, jagged from my gnawing. The envelope is clean and I am slovenly. It is perfect; I am the problem. I long to feel happy when I trace the red heart, but all I see is my dirty fingernail pointing out my sorrow.

The envelope is filled with coupons for me:

Candlelight dinner

Full body massage 1hour

Full body massage 30min

Breakfast in bed

Foot/leg massage 30min

Foot massage 15min

Back massage 15min

Free coupon

I'm going to tear them up and throw them away, because Leon hates, with a lick-the-toilet kind of hate, to give massages. He doesn't want to do it, and after tonight he won't put his love into it. What's the point, when I know he doesn't want to? Even so, I can't bring myself to tear them up. I'm hoping that I can redeem them, save them for when he loves me again.

All this runs through my head as I hold open the door to the fridge in which sits a lemon pie from the restaurant where he first told me he loved me. I don't think he'd say it again if he could go back in time. I close the fridge and think about slicing my wrists, although I'd never do it. Maybe suicide is not about despair. Maybe it's about making someone remember you forever and feel the guilt so that, in a way, you've won.

My black hair swirls across the green velvet couch I've slept on everyday this week. I awake to my name being called. Leon has discovered little food specks in our porcelain toilet, a sign of my failure. Panic inflates my heart but I roll my eyes and don't want to be close to him at all. *Must keep no cash because desire for bad food grows stronger. Must keep heart strong. Must learn new things, not just flounder in the marshmallow goo of my brain.*

*

Shortly after Christmas we decide to move onto a sailboat with the hope of saving money on rent. We'll have to sell most of our things, but the only item I'll be sad to let go is the green velvet couch. For the first time yesterday, I saw our boat, the one my dad thinks is a bad idea for us to buy. But it's too late, because now it's our 36-foot home. The boat is dirty, and the dock is windy and cold. Sometimes I think that if I were back in Hawai'i, I would be happy, even though I know that's a lie. My location is not the problem, I am. Still, I miss the beach, the warm sun, shave ice, and things being familiar. In the harbor our boat sloshes back and forth in the disgusting brown water.

We begin to sell things and pack for the move. Lillie gains strength when I'm stressed. Despite the excitement change brings, it also presses against my nerves. I try to be disciplined, but lately Lillie's voice is too loud and constant. Leon does his best to navigate around the elephant in the room. Every day it's been the same conversation, until today.

Today, Leon starts the same conversation, but this time he breaks down crying and I ask what's wrong. He's been checking everything when he comes home from work: the toilet, the trashcan, the food in the fridge. I want to jump off the roof. He pulls out another letter that tells me how I'm breaking his heart. My mind goes blank and I feel empty, nothing. I've heard this one before.

But this time I'm watching him, in the hollowness of my chest where I hold in the air, and I think, *What am I doing to him? What have I made of him? I never thought I would reduce someone to this. I am selfish. I am pathetic.* And then I feel. I picture him at work, dressed in his coveralls with his name stitched on the front pocket, and I see him turning wrenches, fixing parts on airplanes, putting something back together. I picture him worrying about me all day, about what I'm eating, about what I'm throwing up, and if he'll come home to find me dead on the bathroom floor with a toilet full of wasted food and a body full of wasted life, clutching the porcelain as my heart stops. I picture him crumpling to the floor. I think about how happy we used to be. I think about the phone call he'll need to make to my family. He drove home worrying about me, not knowing what to say or do. He must feel so helpless. I am a bad person, but maybe that's his problem: putting his faith where it doesn't belong—in me.

Dear Christen—

I am writing this letter in an attempt to tell you what I have been feeling lately. I come home everyday and my heart is torn apart from a weakness you have not overcome. I love you so much and have no intentions of not wanting to be with you. I am just hurting by being with you and I don't want you or me to hurt anymore. I need you to get help.

—Leon

I'm killing myself while breaking his heart. I can't stop, but I have to. I have to stop this time.

I stay up late, staring at the ceiling, my eyes bloodshot, fighting the big sleep, the one where I close my eyes and don't wake up. I think Jesus would be sad. I think his eyes would stare through me like piercing swords and slice me right open, and he would know telepathically that I had *not* overcome, so I would not deserve to sit with him. I have not overcome, which implies that I could have, and should have, but I did not.

My body and heart contain the guilt of cities, the guilt of continents, the guilt of worlds. Dear God, where are you when I'm crying, and begging, and pleading for you to save me?

There's something wrong with my stomach. I taught it so well to reject food that now, when I try to be normal, my body rebels and won't let me. The worst feeling isn't pain or discomfort, it's when I know the food is rising, like water in a straw sitting there suspended, waiting in my throat, because my stomach isn't hungry. The worst is waking up throwing up stale lettuce from a late-night dinner that took too long to digest. This is not normal. I'm not normal anymore. I've made my body what I wanted. I beat it into submission, and now out of habit, it rejects. The sadness comes, and with it the searching. *Fill me. Fill me. Give me the taste that I seek.* But nothing does. It's a lost cause. The taste is futile, fleeting, dripping off my tongue. I go crazy, wanting to rip apart the house, knowing the whole time nothing will fill me. Nothing ever does. I'll have to settle for the familiar lost, empty feeling clinking around in my skull, like someone kicking a bottle cap back and forth. I want to be alone, because nothing matters anymore; nothing fills the void. I want to not want anymore.

I can't do this on my own. I need help.

"I found a therapist for you," Leon says. "Her name is Mary."

The air feels heavy and viscous like I'm sucking it in through a straw.

"Will you go and see her?" he asks. "Please?"

I scratch my clavicle and move on to the base of my skull while he waits. I rub my eyes for a while and when I open them he's still there. *Ugh. He isn't going away this time.* "Fine," I say. "I'll go see her. Happy?"

He frowns. "Why do you have to be like that? I'm doing this because I love you."

Whatever. I know he loves me, but why?

4

THE FORTUNE OF THE BLACK HOLE

Each time I get a fortune cookie I save the slip of paper as a prediction for the next phase of my life. This one cracks open and tells me, "Success and happiness will come your way." A second later my phone rings. My insurance provider has approved my request, and I have until the end of the week to voluntarily admit myself to the hospital. I run to the empty alleyway outside the spa where I work and stand there with my back against the concrete wall, squinting in the sun, praying no one decides to take out the trash. Terror/Joy. Like flipping a coin.

I watch my shadow loom before me. I must take a month off from both the coffee shop and the spa without giving a reason. I hate not being honest. That sounds hypocritical, but the disorder is the destructive secret of my life. It is my one locked diary that I will lie about and throw away the key. But God was ready to collect on the deal I'd made with him. *Dear God. If my insurance is accepted, then I'll know you're telling me that I need to go right now and get treatment.* Terror. Joy.

The hospital inpatient program lasts for twenty-eight days. Three days is about my breaking point. The most I've ever done consecutively in the entire eleven years with this disorder was thirty days, and it was an epic battle daily until my defeat. In high school I couldn't even last a day. Every day I would set goals that I'm sure were too rigid, and every time I failed to reach them, I felt like a failure and silently whipped myself with the cruel words I knew by heart. Millions, maybe billions, of words were written in my journals praying to God, asking for help to get through a day with the demons that pinned me and held me down while they laughed at me wriggling there. I struggled to grasp why the God I believed in failed to help me. I finally reached the conclusion that I wasn't doing my part to meet His outstretched hand.

It took Mary less than six therapy sessions to realize I needed round-the-clock help and tell me she was having me admitted to the hospital. My body fought my mind, fought my consciousness like snakes in a pile on the floor rolling over each other. Terror and joy. My whole body resisted but something in my mind whispered, *This may finally make you better.*

When Mary asked me if I was willing to do whatever it took, my mind held onto just the whatever part, not whatever it took, just whatever. My mind said, *No, because they won't make me well. I know it. They'll just make me fat and tell me it's normal and to love my new fat, normal body. They'll try to get me to eat foods that I don't believe in eating, and they'll tell me it's because I have an eating disorder.*

"Do you want to get better?" Mary asked.

"Yes and no," I said. "Yes, I don't want to have this eating disorder. But I won't let them make me fat."

"Do you believe you can recover?"

"No, but I hope I can prove myself wrong." *Dear God, please heal me and make me skinny.*

Two thousand dollars a day is what the hospitalization cost. It's sad, but one of the main reasons I'd never gotten help was because it cost too much money. With the insurance my parents had when I was younger, they still had to pay. When they had first sent me for treatment, at age sixteen, I was anorexic and in denial that anything was wrong. I was on my healthy diet and those stupid people didn't understand how happy I was. They wanted to control me and make me like them. The tiny blonde therapist asked me if I would eat the donut she had on her desk. I said of course I would, if I wanted to eat it, but I didn't want to. I'd thought restriction was willpower. I'd thought that I could eat that donut when I wanted to. It wasn't until later I realized that I could never eat that donut no matter how much I wanted it.

Ever. My refusal to see her again produced a large enough gap in treatment for me to develop bulimia.

At age twenty-two, I went with my brother Zack and a few of his friends to a cliff diving spot where we were all going to jump the three-second free fall into the blue ocean. When I leapt off the rocks, I realized the fall was too far. I panicked, tightened my body, and fell on my back at just the right angle to knock the wind out of me. Coming up from the water, my lungs heaved but no air could get in. Treading water in that brilliant blue ocean, I passed out. If Zack hadn't been there to pull me out, I would have died, and I wouldn't have cared. I wouldn't have cared if I had died.

That afternoon, I sat completely silent in the car as Mom kept asking me what was wrong. I couldn't tell her that part of me wished I had died. Instead, I began to cry, and she didn't know what to do. When she asked if I wanted to see someone, I said, "Yes, take me right now." She drove me immediately to the hospital, and we took the same elevator to the same floor where I had rejected the tiny blonde when I was sixteen. But this time I wanted to die, so I was a little more resigned as we sat in the empty waiting room.

The therapist was a larger lady. There was a bookshelf on the wall and a clock over my head that she watched. Pretty quickly, I decided that she didn't understand me at all, and I began to feed her lies when she asked me questions. She didn't call me on them, and I didn't like that. I asked her if she'd ever had an eating disorder. She said something like, "Let's just focus on you."

What a liar. How can you help me if you won't be honest with me?

When she left the room, I browsed through the books on the bookshelf and read a page about an anorexic girl struggling to eat a whole pear. Pears are fruit, and fruit is healthy for you. I had no problem eating a pear. I was definitely in the wrong place. I stupidly thought I could control myself and that I was in better shape emotionally and therefore didn't need therapy. Going to therapy was admitting weakness.

The therapist watched the clock and ended exactly on time as though there were a buzzer. *OK, now care. OK, now stop.* I wasn't an easy patient. I didn't like her. I wasn't polite. I lied a lot or filled the room with silence. I lasted about four sessions before I knew she couldn't help me, and then I was left alone again.

My dad would say he didn't care how much money it cost for me to get better. But that little voice inside me always said, *If you don't want to get better it's just a waste of his money that you don't deserve.* If I didn't want to get better, he would work and work, day after day, sacrificing his time and his money and his energy just for me to throw it down the drain. Money we didn't have, time you can't get back, energy wasted. I was making everyone's life harder. I was the burden, the one making them struggle. What I wanted was to go away to a place where they didn't have to worry about me and where I wouldn't have to feel guilty. All those years on a seesaw, the voice inside me always won—the voice that told me I didn't want to get well in the end.

"I worry about you." I heard the concern in my dad's voice.

"Don't. That's a burden to me." I heard the bitterness in mine.

And yet through all this, God blessed me with Leon, who is such a good and kind person, with our move to California, with our boat. Why do I flush away all these blessings? It's time to face Lillie. One of us must go, and it will be Leon, Lillie, or me.

Now, for the first time in eleven years, I'm filled with the exhilaration of finally getting help that I am desperate for and terrified of. I know if I don't get help I'll cause more work for myself in the end. I'll twist more knots that I alone will be left to untie. A new little voice has worked its way into my consciousness with a promise: "Success and happiness will come your way." Just like the fortune cookie said. Terror and joy.

5

REASONS I WANT TO GET HELP OR DON'T WANT TO GET HELP

Reasons I want to get help:

1) I hate being controlled by the eating disorder.
2) I can be healthy for Leon.
3) It hinders my life around other people.
4) When people know, I begin to hate them.
5) The eating disorder transforms me into an irritable monster.
6) I know it's not healthy.
7) It's a waste of money.
8) It's a waste of time and ability, and it consumes my thoughts.
9) I can't get better on my own.
10) It hurts my husband and my parents.
11) It may kill me . . . although I'm doubtful (but God's also been protecting me).
12) It's not what God wants for my life.
13) Normal is such a foreign word.
14) Guilt wasted too much of my life already.
15) I don't want to be constantly tortured.
16) It makes me depressed. It's circular. It's only a way to numb feelings.

Reasons I don't want to get help:

1) Deep down I think there is no "better."
2) They just make you fat and call it "better."
3) They control you.
4) When I'm fat, I'm severely depressed, but I'm anti-medication.
5) They won't believe the way I eat is not because of the eating disorder.
6) It's HORRIBLY SCARY.
7) I don't want anyone to know, because then people watch, and I HATE that.
8) How do I tell people, especially my best friend, Julie?
9) People treat you differently once they know.
10) My worst fear is being weak, and this is my biggest weakness.
12) What the fuck is normal anyway?
13) I don't want ANYONE to know.

6

A TASTE OF CONFINEMENT

Today is my last day as this self. Tomorrow I check in to what I hope will be permanent recovery. Scales and mirrors don't terrorize me anymore. What scares me is my rage, the depth of my self-hatred, my superhuman energy that could destroy anything that blocks my way in the moment of binging. I feel no pain. I have one singular focus—food—until the desperation rises up my throat and I have one singular focus—toilet.

Now I will get real help from people I can't evade. I'm excited and scared. Without Mary pushing me, I never would have agreed to being hospitalized, but why the hell is that? It's my life.

I've been thinking about being a little kid, about bike rides and flying kites and making forts. I've been missing my brother and the girl I used to be when we spent entire days rollerblading and jumping speed bumps and eating sandwiches and carrot sticks and grape juice in little waxed paper cups. I miss our forts made of stones and palm tree branches and sitting in the afternoon shade listening to our little blue radio that played a song about getting down on your knees to pray.

I was happy then, without even knowing it. My mind is confined now. Memories of carefree times twist in on themselves with nowhere to go, like roots pushing against a steel box.

I eat my favorite—caramel apple with chocolate—and time ticks closer to the drive to the hospital, to the walk from the car, to the opening of the door, to the terror and the odd excitement that mimics traveling for the first time to a foreign land.

Leon walks me in to the lobby. A nurse comes to greet me. Her hand is cold. I wave goodbye to Leon and try to give him a smile while I grip my suitcase until my fingers hurt. I hold on to my only possessions. My head echoes, *It's been eleven years and you've never been treated.*

I am utterly alone with myself, the person I fear most. What will they do to me? I scan the empty hallways linked with locked doors looming on either side as I follow the nurse. She buzzes us through one gate and then another, as my connection to the world grows dimmer with each robotic sound. A few trees and a square patch of grass give the impression that this may be an afternoon lunch in the park, some false comfort. Straight and to the left, around the pretend park, we pass a large glass window like a fish tank with people inside instead of fish. Every girl notices me as I pass. The girls are all of women's age but I still view us as girls—young and fragile. They stand up or sit higher on the couches, their mouths opening and closing in silence. They scrutinize me with their bubbly eyes, questioning if the nurse will release me into their tank.

In the inside hallway, past the fish tank room, the other nurses look up, purse their lips into smiles, judging if I look like a nice little yes girl. I think they decide I won't be much trouble, so they allow me behind the waist-high swinging door.

I'm taken into the next room, where the shades are pulled down, and I'm asked questions and checked for self-mutilation scars. There are none. I often wonder what my insides look like. Am I rotting away? Was I damaging my body like they said?

"You're not on any medication?" The nurse flips through my paperwork.

"No." I say.

"Nothing to sleep or anything?" She pries as though I'm withholding pertinent information. I shake my head. "No, nothing." She pauses, almost appalled, but regains her composure stuttering, "Well . . . Well, that's good."

"Thanks." I respond to the quasi-compliment and register by her shock that I am quite possibly the only person here who is not on any type of medication. I don't know how to feel about this. For me, pills would be a cop out, the American first step to dealing with anything: let's medicate it. I was used to being depressed. It didn't scare me. Chemically induced happiness, on the other hand, I wouldn't know what to do with that. What's the value of happiness if it's not really mine? It solves nothing.

I'm whisked away for the tour of the unit, where I'm told the rules all the patients must follow. A nurse has to check the toilet before we're allowed to flush. We can take showers only in the mornings before breakfast to prevent us from throwing up in the drains.

"Now you can meet all the girls," the nurse says as we walk towards a door. For a moment I think I might pass out. My mind violently shrieks, and I picture myself screaming and grabbing onto anything in the hallway, so I don't have to go meet the girls. I imagine the nurse screaming too, holding my legs in midair, trying to pull me free.

The nurse knocks on the door, and I realize I'm standing like a good girl next to her in the hallway. I'm taken through the door into the fish tank room where the girls all seem to be around my age. They sit around circular tables with little trays of different foods in front of each of them like hated school lunches. All fish eyes look up. My presence feels huge, as though they'd actually heard my blood-curdling scream in the hallway. All eyes fixate in my direction. I stand perfectly still, like prey, hearing my heart tick like the clock on the wall.

"You can have a seat here," the nurse says, and everything begins to move again.

Some girls go back to their food, while others keep watching me with interest. The interested ones size me up, trying to figure out whether I'm anorexic or bulimic. They're smug because I'm vulnerable and brand new and terrified, and they know it. In this room, I'm exposed instantly, and without a sound, everyone knows my deepest secret: I have an eating disorder. Just the same, without a word, I know theirs.

I'm just in time for check-in, the nurse tells me, and she points to the wall where a large sign with black letters reads:

GOALS

Goal: Morning

3 positive affirmations

Yes or no?

- *Suicide*
- *AWOL*
- *Self-harm (includes binging, purging, restricting thoughts)*

How do you feel?

- *Physically*
- *Emotionally*
- *Spiritually*

0-10 (best to worst)

- *Anxiety*
- *Safety*

Goal: Evening

Did you meet your goal?

I'm told to say my name.

"Hi, I'm Christen," I say.

"Hi, Christen," is the immediate response, all in unison like weird, brainwashed girls of a summer camp. Most people don't look up from their tables. They're obviously bored with the routine. I'm relieved the nurse lets me skip the affirmations, because I don't know what they are and don't want to ask in front of everyone. She asks me to give three words that describe how I'm feeling.

"Perturbed, vulnerable, blasé." This is enough for now, but I feel my heart drumming as the attention shifts to someone else. The drill is finished after all of us have had a turn to speak. Then the dinner trays are stacked on a wheeling cart after the nurse nods that each person has eaten everything. A tiny, fragile girl brings up her tray, but the nurse shakes her head. She can't eat anymore, she says. She's almost in tears, so I look away, embarrassed to witness the intimate moment when she crumples in her chair and drops her tray back down on her table. All I can see is her long, straight blonde hair falling down the back of her oversized black sweatshirt. She's staring at the food, unmoving, fixed, ignoring us all.

There's one older lady in the group who is tall and gangly and comes right up to me to show me around the room. My gratitude is immense. Silent and astute, I, the perfect student, follow her as she pulls out the cabinet drawers. "This is where we keep the glue sticks to make collages. And here are the forms you have to fill out for meals. I'll show you how to do that later. I've been here for a few weeks. I used to be fat—268 pounds—and I decided to have gastric bypass surgery." She fingers the stacks of magazines shoved into one drawer. "Everyone has to make a collage when they're here, so here are all the magazines you can choose from." My eyes scan the covers as she continues, "My stomach was only the size of a thumb, so I'd overeat on accident and throw up, but then I began purging on purpose, followed by restricting until I almost died. Do you know how many starches and fats you've been assigned?" I shake my head. She has white skin that hangs just a little from reaching that age when the elastin and collagen start to give up. Her eyebrows are black and furry with a little worm of hair crawling from one brow to the other.

My room has three plain hospital beds and an armoire-style dresser with two doors that open from the center. A blue flannel blanket and a clean pillowcase folded and waiting on the ends of each of the two empty beds remind me of airplane pillows and blankets that tease you with their smallness. I'm starting to get a headache from all the florescent lights. A waxy green apple in my bag might fend off my headache, but I'm told I have to wait for it to be approved before I can eat it. Even when I tell them I'll sit in the chair and they can watch me eat it, they refuse. I don't want to throw up my apple. I'm asking to eat it. This seems like a no-brainer. I doubt their ability to take care of me if they cannot even fathom logic.

In my room, the nurse goes through all my belongings. "We have a no string policy," she informs me as she begins to take away all my things. "I'll need to take that," she says, picking up my sweatpants.

"Why?" I ask in a tone that implies she's an idiot.

"The drawstring," she answers as though I should have known. "Your shoes, same reason, unless you want to take the laces off?"

I look at her thinking she must be joking. Shoelaces are somewhat vital to a shoe. She's not joking.

"Okay then," she throws my shoes on the left side of the bed, the contraband side, "You can't have the earphones, any device to play music, or these tweezers." (I guess my roommate's caterpillar eyebrows will have to stay). She announces everything out loud as if to mock me as she takes it away. "Cotton swabs, dental floss, batteries, and plastic bags."

Am I that stupid to try to kill myself with cotton swabs and dental floss? Now that practically everything I brought is on the contraband side of the bed, she marks all my things on her clipboard and puts them in my suitcase, which I'm also not allowed to have. I hate being controlled, but I stay silent even though I feel like telling her that I can't wait to be naked, dirty, and bored for twenty-eight days. I want to bet her that someone can still commit suicide with a T-shirt or a pair of underwear, but I stay silent because I want my underwear. What are they going to do to me here that they fear me having items like a battery?

Since she's taken away all my plastic bags, all my remaining stuff is laid out across the bed, so she can log my meager possessions, go through my wallet, and count my rings. I'm now in prison, and this is only hour one of twenty-eight days of hell. I stare down at my red, laceless shoes and want to cry.

It is agreed that I'm allowed to eat my apple only if I promise to eat my snack later. *Well, thank you very much, since I'm hungry now.* In view of the nurse, I try to make the crunch extra loud. I'm doing a good job as it echoes through my head, the suction pull when each chunk finally rips free, but I fear I'm accomplishing nothing, like angrily pressing the button to hang up a cell phone. *Take that.*

I have to stop chewing to hear as she goes over the meal plan and the choices of what I can eat tomorrow.

"You're very calm about all this," she says.

Teeth sink in, suctioned rip, loud crunch. *Screw you.* My eyes glance up from the menu. "I don't think it's healthy to eat that much food," I respond in a monotone. I stare at the food list while anxiety fills me and swells my throat. The list shows that tomorrow they're going to make me eat snacks like teddy bear-shaped cinnamon crackers, which are junk food. If I refuse to eat something, I'm told they'll substitute the absent calories with a calorie shake. Inside, I'm freaking out. Outside, I try to remain dull, like I don't give a shit, like they don't scare me.

I have never been so tired after eating one small green apple. I head towards the fish tank, where I sink into the couch, trying to make myself invisible, then glance around the room and take my own survey of the people. The small blonde girl from earlier catches my interest immediately because I've felt her despair, staring at food that my anxiety would not let me eat. She's thin and reminds me of myself when I was anorexic.

Even though I know the torture it required to maintain my 97-pound body, I use anorexia as my goal to get back to. It sounds so much nicer to say, "I undereat," rather than, "I stuff myself until I'm disgusted and then vomit it all back up."

When I was anorexic, my life was regimented. I woke up early, ran a certain number of miles, monitored every bite I ate. It took a toll, mentally, all the things I had to do, but at least I felt somewhat in control. At least I had rules to follow, and if I succeeded, I deemed myself somewhat good. When I switched over to bulimia I was never good, because I was never in control. With anorexia I wouldn't—couldn't—eat the cookie, no discussion, but with bulimia I agonized over it, justified it, ate it, hated myself, threw it up, wanted more, hated myself more. It was an endless cycle of shame. With anorexia, I felt somewhat healthy, I exercised, I had goals. Bulimia felt like giving up, like why bother at all?

I say that I was tricked out of anorexia. People noticed that I was getting thinner, and I was mortified in public when anyone asked me about food. I hated how the attention put a spotlight on me, and I was becoming exhausted from following my own rules. I missed food. I missed desserts, and if I wanted to eat them I had to get rid of them somehow. At first, bulimia was only for the desserts. However, once I realized I could get rid of one thing, why not more? Then, I began to gain weight no matter how much I threw up.

My value as an anorexic person was based on my level of self-control. After bulimia hooked me, my value shrank to nothing, because I constantly teetered one bite away from a fall. Anorexia, which gave me control and a thinner body, was an oddly appealing antidote when life was constant chaos.

The thing that made me different as an anorexic was that I never skipped meals, so I got to reward myself with food and punish myself with exercise. I was an athlete in high school. I could run on my lunch breaks, have my lunch alone in the locker room, practice basketball for two to three hours after school, and go home to eat a small dinner. It didn't seem strange to think of my body as a type of machine. I was fine-tuning it, making it work better. The pride I felt when I refused to eat junk food is what became the addiction. People remarked on my willpower, and the pride in me would swell because, yes, I was so good and strong and diligent and focused and perfect. *Thank you for noticing.*

Instead of trying to hide how skinny I was, I avoided people at school and didn't make any close friends. Why would I act like an anorexic and wear baggy clothes to hide my accomplishments?

When I fell into bulimia, things changed. I started to camp out in the library and dress for Alaskan weather. I still wanted to be left alone, but the bulimia made me ashamed of myself. At least with the anorexia I was proud.

The summer before my freshman year of high school, I was fifteen, and I worked as a junior lifeguard at the pool. At lunchtime, when the doors closed to the public, the head lifeguard would make us swim laps, and I had a paper-thin black suit that made me feel sleek like a fish.

That summer my dad found out he had high cholesterol and my mom stopped buying red meat.

Another junior lifeguard noticed how much we loved desserts, but we bet that we could stop eating them for a month. I joked with people that I was on a diet, as I pinched the half-inch of fat on my tummy. After the first week, the other lifeguard had given up and was back to eating cookies, but I had a goal in my head and I'd already won, so that made me feel powerful. If a little victory made me feel good, wouldn't a bigger one be better?

When school started, my ID photo showed my teeth blinding white against the dark tan of my skin. When lunchtime came around, I was so used to swimming laps that it felt weird not to be exercising, so I began to run in the ravines and neighborhoods behind the school. At first I felt energized, but soon it became something I needed to do, a compulsion that I thought about and dreaded during all the classes leading up to lunch. *Just run all around Mânoa and then your mind will be quiet, and I won't bother you about it anymore,* the voice said.

During that year I was furious with my mom because she constantly tried to feed me. Every morning she made English muffins with jam or waffles with little pieces of banana in the shape of a happy face. Morning smoothies were a daily ritual, most likely her attempt to get me to consume more calories. We had dinners together as a family, and I became accustomed to the tension and anxiety I felt as I pushed food around my plate, so things wouldn't touch each other. I had started out trying to be healthy, and before I knew it, I was the one making up insane little games I had to win or else my anxiety would shoot through the roof. At night I watched the light from my parents' TV flickering in their bedroom as I sat in the darkness of the living room maniacally doing sit-ups and recounting everything I'd eaten.

Freshman year I looked like Alicia Silverstone in *Clueless*. I wore pleated skirts and black knee-high socks and berets. I wanted to be like her character in the movie, untouchable and outspoken and fun, but I was shy and socially inept and could feel my face flush bright red each time the guy I liked talked to me in class.

Every clique I walked by in the quad on my way to the locker room tested my ability to pretend I wasn't freaking out inside. "Don't talk to me don't talk to me, don't talk to me," I'd pray under my breath. *Because if you talk to me, then you'll know I'm weak and fragile and you can crack me right open. I'd like you to think I'm strong. I'd like to give you the illusion I'm unapproachable. Don't talk to me, don't talk to me, please, don't talk to me.*

My parents had no idea what to do, because I kept silent and smiled pretty and pretended that I was happy. Even in my journals I wrote in cryptic metaphors, because I was afraid someone would read them, that my privacy would be invaded. When my parents got angry or confronted me about my eating or exercising, I shrugged it off with a joke or ignored them completely.

Then, one day towards the end of my freshman year, I had a rare moment of letting down my guard. It started with my dad's favorite question, the one I loathed because I had to lie: "Are you happy?"

I was sitting on the couch in our living room.

"Who do you eat lunch with?" my dad asked.

In that moment, my heart hurt too much, and I cracked and began to sob. "I eat lunch alone every day in the locker room."

Tears filled my mom's eyes. "What about Julie? Can't you eat with her?"

"She doesn't have any of my same breaks," I said. My dad was worried. I could feel it.

Why did you break down? Weak. Baby. Why are you worrying them?

They tried to tell me what to do, because they loved me and didn't want to see their child become a crumpled crying skinny mess on their couch.

"Why don't you try to go to the cafeteria and find someone to eat with?" my dad asked. "I'm sure you can do that."

I stopped crying. With new resolve, I could probably do what he suggested. It was a huge step, but I told myself I'd try because I was so sad inside.

The next day, I felt six years old instead of sixteen. My heart beat wildly, and I was scared and happy, risking it all by stepping up the hill. The clear doors of the cafeteria beckoned as I clutched my green plastic lunchbox and looked around. But no one was there except for a small group of kids I had never seen. I felt my heart sink and lock into a hard ball in my chest. I was alone.

As I walked back to the locker room, I felt foolish. Every day after that, I walked straight to the locker room to bypass the hurt, because if I chose to be alone at least I was in control. I didn't have to risk other people hurting me. After that, I mastered pretending I was happy and lied so the truth wouldn't hurt my parents.

"Are you happy?" my dad asked.

No. No. No. No. No. Smile. "Yes," I'd say and change the subject.

*

The little blond girl that reminds me of me is in her own world making a collage. Her back facing me, her baggy black sweatshirt pooling down to her thumbs as her little fingers busy themselves with paper scraps, she ignores everyone around her in the room, putting out that same untouchable vibe I had. I wonder if she, too, had a lunchbox that once held hope.

One girl is watching me from the other side of the couch, and finally I look up.

"What are you?" she asks me point-blank. I stare back at her as she explains, "Anorexic? Bulimic?"

This is the first time I have ever told anyone. My mind skips a beat, and I grasp for answers, knock back the impulse to hide or defend myself, because, *hello,* she already knows. I grapple with what to say. Anorexic sounds nicer, cleaner, prettier, and if people see you eating, then they think you're OK. Bulimia on the other hand is dirty, gross, retched, and people watch you all the time. You are never clear of their eyes, their judgment, their knowing.

"Bulimic," I say, because why not face the fact that I'm not bone thin and anorexic anymore except in my own mind.

"Me, too," she says and scoots closer to me as if this bonds us. I let out a small breath because I'm almost happy she's bulimic. Now she won't judge me.

Everyone wolfs down the snack as though it were their last meal and they were starving and being timed for a grand prize. Later I discover it's what they do just to get the food down so they don't have to think about what they're eating. The nurse hands me pretzels, which I didn't choose, and I'm pissed. She tells me no, that I can't have peanut butter like one of the other girls and no, I can't have anything else for that matter, which sucks because I never willingly eat foods I know I'll automatically want to throw up, pretzels being on that long list. This is one of the various screwed-up rules that eating disorder patients make for ourselves. We put foods into categories, label them safe or not safe—the same rules that define our happiness, our lives, our sanity. The strange thing about the rules is that they follow no set pattern or structure and every patient's rules are different.

When I become friends with the girl in the black sweatshirt, and she tells me that every time I ate a peanut butter and jelly sandwich, she nearly had a heart attack because I was eating fat, sugar, and carbs all at once, which broke all of her counting rules. However, a peanut butter and jelly sandwich was one of the few foods I considered safe—"safe" because I wouldn't want to throw it up.

My pretzels suck, and I play with them the way a child at the dinner table fiddles with some hated vegetable, the difference being I am going to have to eat them no matter what. Then I remember I can have a shake instead, so I opt for the chocolate one, wishing I'd chosen it in the first place. *Maybe I can drink all my meals in chocolate,* I think happily.

The nurse must see my smile and read my thoughts because she squashes the hope quickly. "You cannot drink your meals. You have to eat all your food. If you don't, we give you the shake to supplement the extra calories."

Whatever.

My side hurts as I brush my teeth and put on my socks. I have a drawstring on my pants the nurse didn't catch. I am giddy with this knowledge. *I have contraband. Ha, ha. What the hell do you expect me to do with a drawstring? Wrap it around my neck and pull?*

*

I hate them! They lied to me when they took my phone. They said they'd give it back, so I could call Leon. Now they say no, that once I check in my phone, it's not my property anymore. But I have to use a phone to call Leon to give him the number to this stupid place. I need to be able to call my parents and Julie. I normally call them daily, and if they don't hear from me it will raise suspicion.

As I'm carrying all my stuff to the bathroom, a nurse stops me and takes my blood pressure and temperature and gives me a cup to pee in. I've been awake for less than two minutes. I hate this place.

Wash face. Brush teeth. The shower rooms are small white cubicles and remind me of being underground. I keep imagining the showers where they locked the Holocaust victims and turned on the gas. There are no windows. The floor is cold, hard, white two-by-two-inch tiles. My cubicle has a shower curtain and my things keep sliding off the plastic bench as if the room were tilted. The temperature gauge for the water is near the door, while the actual shower is at the far side of the room, so I have to keep getting out and fiddling with the knob. I'm half wet and freezing. If I plan it right, I probably can do some leg lifts or running in place without being caught.

After my shower adventure, they still refuse to give me my phone. They point to the two yellow pay phones outside the eating disorder room, but I need a phone card to call out, and I don't have one.

"What should I do?" I ask them. "Should I call my husband with my nonexistent phone card to tell him I need him to get me a phone card so I can call him?"

They point to the yellow phones. What about this situation is so hard for them to understand? Finally, I'm left with the choice to either yell at their incompetence or cry angrily in my room, which, I tell myself, is the wiser option.

While I'm crying, my roommate slides through the door and sits on the edge of my bed to listen. I rant about how much I need to make a call, because if I don't, people will start asking questions. If I can lie to my parents and best friend for twenty-eight days while I'm here, then I can keep this all a secret and they won't know how messed up I've become. The caterpillar on her brow does a shake, and she says I should tell my family because withholding the truth is detrimental to my recovery. *Ugh.*

They weigh us before breakfast as I stand tall in the hospital gown, and I'm almost sure I see the digital numbers say 122. How did I get fatter overnight? Didn't I weigh 120 or less before I came in here? I'm told from now on, I'll get weighed backwards, so only they can monitor my progress. What the hell does progress mean? Are they trying to make me gain weight? I don't need to gain any weight. When I'm throwing up, bulimic, I weigh more because of the binging. They can't be making me gain, can they?

Breakfast comes. We eat all our meals together in the fish tank room seated around our tables. The fish tank is where we spend most of our days. At every breakfast and dinner, we each have to introduce ourselves and go through our goals lists. It's stupid, but I might as well get used to it, because we'll do it every morning and evening for the next twenty-eight days.

Silently, I swirl my apple, peanut butter, soymilk, and cereal together. This sucks. I want to meet with the nutritionist. My eyes try to focus on my bowl but wander to the girl's tray across the table. She's eating enough food to be a binge for me. My heart is pounding. *She's half my size. Doesn't anyone see how much food they're making her eat?*

It's my turn to speak. "My name is Christen," I say, distracted.

"Hi, Christen," everyone drones.

"Three things about yourself you want to be true or are true."

"I am lucky to have food to eat," I say.

"Yes, you are," everyone answers. That's always the response.

"No. No. No. Yes." *Suicide, AWOL, contracts, binge/purge thoughts.* "Physically, I'm feeling full, tense, and I have a headache. Emotionally, I'm frustrated and angry. Spiritually, I'm lost. Safety: zero. Anxiety: five. My goal for the day is to eat and not feel tortured by wanting to throw up."

The others take their turns, and I begin to like what people say about what they want to be true. "I am safe. I am happy. I love my body." These things make me sad, though, because I know we all want to believe them but don't.

Group therapy begins as everyone scrambles for the best, most comfortable seats around the circle. I wait, so I don't take anyone's seat and make them mad.

Jackie, one of the therapists who runs the programs, introduces herself and says we'll be sharing collages today. She's has ice blue eyes, soft wavy black hair that falls down past her shoulders, and an I-mean-business attitude that leaves no room for anyone to interrupt her.

The doctor who oversees my treatment pulls me out into the hallway and tries to convince me to consider taking meds. I tell him I'll think about it, knowing I won't.

Finally, I meet the nutritionist, who is a big-boned lady with a dirty blonde bob cut. She wears a business suit with heels that click down the hallway as she makes her way to me. She assigns me a ridiculous number of starches. My eyes can only stare at the numbers she writes on my paper. Most starches are binge foods and clog the intestines, which means they must be thrown up. I now hate her as well. Her black ballpoint pen writes, *I'm better than you,* but when I look again it says, *7 starches, 7 proteins, 3 veg, 2 fruit, 2 milk, 2 fat.*

I attempt to tell her that I'm a vegan and that I don't eat protein or drink milk. She stares at me as though I'm trying to finagle my way out of eating. *This is bullshit.* I would never drink that much milk. I mean, I like soymilk but two cups? And seven starches is just frickin' ridiculous. I may have two pieces of bread all day as my only starches, and they expect me to eat seven. No way. How is this supposed to help me when I will never ever eat like this at home when I leave?

The only thing about today that begins to look good is a nice nurse who lets me send a fax to Leon telling him the number to call me on the pay phone.

Later that night he calls.

"Christen." A girl yells down the hallway and plunks the phone on the countertop. Leon and I have a three-way call with my mom, and I feel more at peace despite headaches that have gotten progressively worse. Leon tells me he's written me two letters, and he hates to write. It makes me want to get better for him, so he can have someone to grow old with. Hanging up the phone severs my tie to the outside world. Click. Loneliness.

After dinner and snack, I finally get to talk to a few of the girls, and we share a few laughs about our personal favorite binge foods. We devise a fake menu, which helps me feel glad I'm with people who understand my deepest secret. We laugh about our fake menu items of six cupcakes with globs of frosting and a pot full of macaroni and cheese.

When I'm happy, I feel a tinge of hope for a future with Leon and perhaps growing old with him. My brother and I used to tell our parents we were going to live only until forty and die before our bodies began to break down. Maybe I'll add on a few more years.

7

WHY WE HATE GOD

Wash face, brush teeth, get vitals checked. I'm told I now can keep my cotton swabs in my room, so they must think I'm a good patient. I'm stumped about what damage I could do with a cotton swab other than poke out my eardrum, an unappealing thought. Then I'd be the bulimic half-deaf girl, and they would surely take my cotton swabs away.

After breakfast we recite the goals, which is starting to feel like a game.

"I'm Christen."

"Hi, Christen."

I'm beginning to like this, and I experiment with how loud I can agree with people before the nurse thinks I'm being wise.

Funny thing is, I have lots of so-called friends at home, but none know I have an eating disorder. My support list has only one name: Leon. The reason my parents aren't on my list, even though they know I have an eating disorder, is because they're always making me feel guilty, like I'm so much better and smarter and more intelligent than this disorder, so why can't I just get over it? No, they are not good supports. Sometimes I don't think Leon is either. He tries so hard, but it comes down to me being able to tell him how to help me and then accepting his help. If I don't know how to help myself, what the hell do I tell him? And even if I knew what I needed, I'm not sure how to ask for it.

The group claps for one of the girls who is leaving the hospital today and makes comments about how well thought-out her home-care plan is. Then

Jackie, allows one of the patients to read her angry letter. "Who is the angry letter addressed to?" Jackie wants to know. "God," she says flatly and opens her black and white composition notebook.

"Dear God." Her words come out soft and hard, hitting the floor with her confusion and loneliness, and filled with so many questions. She feels God and the church abandoned her when she was raped and rumors spread that she was a slut. "And where were you, God?" she says, when she was being beaten until she couldn't breathe. "Where were you, God, when it hurt so bad?" How could He allow this when she was praying to Him about these things? She was told she couldn't hate God. Now she says with such conviction, "But I do hate you, God. I hate you."

The room is silent. I'm crying, and I can't respond or see that she's crying, too. The room is a blur. Her words remind me how I rebelled against God because I couldn't feel anything. I wanted Him to punish me just so I could feel something, to know He was there. Those feelings linger like a whisper in fog. I'd walk into clubs feeling beautiful and bitter and angry and loving the sense of power it gave me.

It's as though God has abandoned both of us. Where was God when we needed him?

I hear her voice as it cracks. I hear her broken hope. We believed in a God that didn't save us. This is why we cry. This is why we hate God. We hate God because we once loved Him. We hate God because we believed He could hear us. We hate Him because even through all our pain, when feeling forsaken, we know deeper in our hearts that He's there and that He loves us, and we hate Him because we can't stop believing in Him.

*

The dietician picked out my lunch, which is way too much food for me. I'm not even halfway through when I feel it involuntarily coming up, and I have to swallow. I swallow all my annoyance, anger, and resentment, hoping the dietician will trip down the stairs to her bloody death.

*

My therapist introduces herself as Margaret, when I seat myself in her office across the hall from the scales where they will weigh me backwards. She's a little shorter than I and has brownish blonde hair and pouty lips, and her eyes seem to contain years of other people's pain. Something about how she talks makes me feel safe, and I find myself telling her everything from the beginning, from that summer I was fifteen. It comes out easily because I've analyzed it so many times.

"I was tricked into bulimia. In my family, everyone ate. My mom woke up early to make us breakfast and pack us all lunches, which Zack and I took to school and my dad took to work. After work, she would sometimes bring me snacks before basketball practice—veggie maunapua or mochi or some sort of sandwich from her job at the yacht club.

"Every night we had dinners together at the table, all four of us. When I was anorexic, I still ate but I developed weird ways of eating. Eating became an art, picking apart small sections, cutting things into little bites, making sure nothing touched even a drop of fat. People watching me made me nervous, and I preferred to eat alone. For a whole year I didn't eat a single dessert, until one night, my mom baked a pan of date bars, and I inhaled a whole row of them before I could stop myself. *Fat, fat, fat, fat, fat pig* was all I heard all night. My anxiety was at a level ten. How could I have let my perfect façade slip? Even the miles I ran during lunch the next day didn't give me any peace about what I'd done. After that, I determined I was becoming depressed because now it was no longer about being healthy. My mind wouldn't let me eat the things I wanted without screaming and belittling me into submission."

"So what did you do?" Margaret asks.

"Well… one afternoon everything changed. I met Lillie."

Margaret furrows her eyebrows trying to keep up, "Who is Lillie?"

"The name I gave to my eating disorder—the voice in my head. Anyway, our neighbor had a party. A big fat piece of chocolate cake ended up on a plate in my hand, and I ran with it all the way down the stairs, home to my empty house. I stood in my living room and stuffed a bite of the chocolate into my mouth. But I couldn't swallow. I just couldn't accept the calories, so

I let it roll around my mouth and spit it out in the napkin. I could finally taste chocolate I'd been missing for a year. That night I wrote in my journal, 'I have discovered a way to eat and not be fat.'

"Did the spitting continue for long?"

"No. There was no space for me to eat and spit, even though I desperately wanted to eat desserts again without having to pay the price. The problem was we lived in a 500-square-foot house, my brother and I shared a room, and from anywhere in the house you could see everywhere else. The only place with any privacy was the bathroom, and since we had only one, longer stays were met with frantic knocks on the door. 'I gotta go now,' my brother would say. 'I'm turtle-heading.'"

"OK…" Margaret's eyes open wide. She has long bangs that make her look as though I'm talking to someone my own age. "Continue…"

"Yeah, in our house, even privacy was a thing to be shared, and we were a close loving family because of it."

Margaret smiles sadly like she wants to protect me from something. "Do you remember the first time you made yourself throw up?"

I nod.

She waits, leaning forward in expectation. She reminds me of a pretty baby calf I'd seen in Costa Rica with the most innocent eyes, capable of pulling out all my secrets with their goodness.

"On a peaceful school night when I had been anorexic for about a year. My willpower against sweets was dwindling. My mom had made a chocolate pudding pie with a graham cracker crust. I'm not sure if I ate it knowing I was going to try throwing up or if I just ate the dessert and freaked out right after, but I excused myself and, while my family talked inside, I stood five feet from the front door with one hand braced against the wooden post that held up our porch roof and the other making myself gag. I heaved and forced myself to do it again until I could taste chocolate, and I tipped over like a teapot and threw up into the plants below. As soon as dinner started coming up, I stopped."

"You didn't throw up everything?" she asks with a hint of interest.

"I wanted to keep the good food in. I just didn't want the calories from the dessert."

She nods like this makes absolute sense. I decide I like her.

"After taking a few breaths and drawing in my tears, I went back inside to my smiling family."

"So how did your parents finally find out?"

"Well, I didn't want to keep gagging and having my eyes water, because I hated the feeling, so after a few days I knew I could be better. I was a straight-A student, so I used my mind and knew that I could will my stomach to turn, and I did. It was magic. No finger, no gagging, just lean over and voilà, presto-chango, dessert in a bush. After about two weeks of me going outside after dinner, my dad discovered the rotting plant. How stupid. I'd been throwing up into a plant in front of the porch expecting no one to notice. There were bits of green beans in the dirt. He called me into his room, and I lied to his face."

"How did that feel?"

"I was so angry and numb. I just stood there in a silent standoff. His eyes were like spider webs. I asked if I could go and he shrugged, so I left the house. I intended to throw up, but first I wanted to pet the neighbor's rabbit. We shared a garage with our neighbors, and they kept their rabbit in a cage near the cars. I tried to spend time with it so it wouldn't feel alone. As I bent down to the cage I heard my mom call me. I couldn't leave the house without someone following me and having to know where I was.

"What did you want?" Margaret asks.

"I wanted to disappear forever. I sounded like Satan when I finally answered, 'What?'

"She said, 'How long are you going to stay up here?' She was worried.

"I said, 'I don't know.' I know I sounded hard. I didn't feel any remorse. I thought, *Just get the hell away from me.*

"She stood behind me as I petted the rabbit through the cage. I wanted her to disappear. I concentrated all my hate in a sharp spike and shot it outwards through the skin on my back.

"She said, 'You're not going to throw up, are you?' like it was her fault.

"I almost screamed, but I had been thinking about throwing up. I gritted my teeth until they hurt. I told her, 'Go away.'"

I remember feeling my words hit my mom like they hurt. I block the emotional part of the memory and continue speaking matter-of-factly. "She let out a small breath like people do before they cry, and she walked away. I tilted my head down to peer under the car and watched her slippers shuffle away until she was gone."

"And then?" Margaret says.

"My legs hurt from squatting, so I sat next to the rabbit cage and breathed out all the hatred into the garage. That was the night I knew I was going to have to start throwing up in the toilet, and I would have to teach myself to be almost silent, because I knew they were listening a few feet away in the living room. The only thing separating the bathroom from the living room was a plywood door that was less than half an inch thick."

Margaret watches me push my Italian hands under my legs, so I'll stop talking with them. This is the most I have ever told anyone in my life. I'm spilling out in all directions like a water bomb.

"From that day on, Lillie was there, and my life was never the same, because what started out as throwing up only desserts gave way to throwing up any other food I wouldn't allow myself to have, which was nearly everything. The rest of the years of high school blur into one big wait for my family to go away and do some activity I refused to do. I'd feel massive anger and anxiety as they lagged until the last minute. I'd try to remain all smiles while I wanted to scream, 'Get out of the house!' Up the stairs they'd go, and I'd wait to hear if they were gone and then out would come the food in piles. I raided the refrigerator like someone who hadn't eaten in years. I was always watching the clock, waiting for the sound of their steps, terrified when not all the food would come up."

"What was that like for you?" I can hear in Margaret's voice that she really cares.

"Constant paranoia. I feared I'd get caught, that my parents would come home early. But the worst fear was that I didn't get all the food back up, that some of it had already sunk to the bottom of my stomach where I couldn't throw up enough to get to. Nothing ever filled me, and my life became one long strand of moments before I was alone again with my food. It was worse than anorexia in lots of ways. So much more violent. So much more anger, and the cravings never stopped. On top of that, I got fatter and paler and my face swelled. All of me was revolting. As much as I tried, once bulimia had me, it never let me go back to being a nice, silent anorexic girl."

"Have you ever thought about getting treatment before?"

"I thought about it, but then I'd convince myself I didn't need it. I did the yo-yo. Lillie became a quasi-friend, so I always kept her close enough to reach for if I wanted her or she wanted me."

"When did you first think about getting treatment?"

"When I had my side pain. My junior year of college, I studied abroad in Germany. Two of my friends and I went traveling for six weeks in Europe before I went to Germany. I didn't work out at all, my knees were out of shape, and I blew them both out on my first run. My knees were shot. I could barely walk, let alone exercise, so when my luggage arrived and I couldn't fit into my jeans, panic and horror set in. I spent the night sobbing on the floor of my room. The binges were more severe because I had to hold the food in longer and longer, all the way home on the bus, and my intestines stopped working. I could no longer use the bathroom."

"Did you go to the doctor?"

"Yes, and they didn't find anything. But I thought I deserved it, you know, like I was finally getting my punishment. Everything that was stuck inside me formed a tight ball like a fist that pushed constantly against my left side. I began to think I was walking tilted to the left. I drank liters of prune juice that came out the same way it went in but with nothing more. This was it. I had succeeded in killing my body, and now I was going to pay the price. Looking back on that time scares me, because I honestly thought I was going to die in my bedroom in Germany and my life would have been such a waste. Lying in bed at night I could hear my heart thud through my body like a monster trying to push free. The dizziness would overtake me. I'd beg God to heal me. I'd get out of bed and draft a letter to my Dad—an apology for being me—in case I died in my sleep. Then I'd lie down and keep reviewing the mental list of consequences:

What if I damaged my kidney? (I need that. It's, like, a vital organ.)
What if I herniated my stomach?
What if my heart got lurched from its proper place?
Why is there a lump in the center of my chest? That's not normal.
What if I will never be able to eat again?
What if this pain in my side is forever?
What if I damaged my heart and that's why I hear it?
What if it's too late?

"In Germany, I was convinced I was going to die and I was to blame."

Margaret leans over and frowns. Her lips tilt down like taffy round the edges.

"I didn't want to use laxatives, but no one could find anything physically wrong with me, so I waited until I could go home to the doctors in Hawai'i. After an array of tests, they told me they could find nothing wrong and that perhaps it was all in my mind. I smiled politely and shot them eight times in my head before I walked away.

"The pain lasted over a year. I am not making this up. It would be there if I didn't eat, and it got worse when I did. Food became my enemy. I hardly ate at all, but I didn't lose any weight, and I was still lethargic, tired, and dizzy sometimes. I just wanted to die, so the pain would end."

"What made it finally go away?"

"I don't know," I say, baffled. "One day, over a year later, for no reason at all, it began to dissipate, until all that was left was my terror of food, because food equaled pain. I also met a guy, Leon. We'd fallen in love. I was happy for the first time in years."

"That's all we have time for today," Margaret says softly with her sad smile.

The walls are ghost white as I walk down the hall, my body pulsing, knowing I like her, and hoping she can explain why I do this to myself and how I can deal with it. At least I feel like she's on my side. I've never felt like someone who wanted me to get better was on my side. It has always felt like they were trying to control me, but Margaret is different. She listens to me. I've never met a therapist before who looked at me patiently, without judgment, with no agenda. She pays attention. It reminds me of that cow in Costa Rica. I held its gaze and whispered to it everything I was thinking because I was afraid talking would be too loud. And it watched me, blinking, absorbing every word. People are rarely grounded. When they are it's surprising and a little unnerving. If they sit there unmoving, staring at me, actually caring, I will eventually tell them everything. She is safe. She is unflinching. She is with me, not trying to control me. She is just with me.

*

"Why?" is the question as we sit around on the cluster of couches in the fish tank room. "If I'm so smart, why do I kill myself? If I'm so smart, why can't I convince myself to stop?" I think group therapy is bullshit. They say food is the tool, just the Band-Aid to cover up the issue behind it. So what is the issue? They say we're here because it forces us to take food out of the equation so that we can deal with the deeper things we're trying to suppress with the food. They say it's a numbing out tool. I think they lie. I like to eat. I don't want to get fat, so I throw up. When I binged, I never used to throw up *everything*, just enough so that I wasn't full. In a sense it still seems justifiable. In a sense it seems OK. They tell us to think of our triggers. I throw up because I want to be thinner. They tell me to look deeper.

There's a deeper?

After group and until dinner we're left on our own in the fish tank. Ellie, the blond girl I noticed on the first day, who reminds me of me when I was anorexic, goes to sleep, but I can't shut off my mind, so I decide to cut up magazines and start on my collage. My stomach feels like someone's sprouting seeds in it. My abdomen is in pain, bloating as my body mixes up the food inside. The sound of scissors tearing through the pages cuts the air—fragmenting time, removing the past, removing the future until, for a moment, all that's left is right now.

But my mind drifts back to Margaret's question, "Tell me about your family?"

Just the memory of that question rekindles my annoyance. It was so

Freudian. There's nothing wrong with my family. I had a great childhood, and, as much as I like her, I can't understand why Margaret's so determined to break my world apart.

8

SCREW THEM

He told people I'm in the hospital. Leon told his grandparents I have an eating disorder and I'm in the hospital. He outed me. How dare he? I am pissed beyond belief. I am terrified of anyone knowing, and all I can think of is food—all the things I would binge on in this moment.

I have been betrayed. I feel exposed, lied to, pried open. My worst fear was just handed to me as a gift. I am in a rage.

I'm trying to ask myself why it's so bad if people know. *Because it just is!*

In my room, I'm pacing, trying to burrow holes in the floor, so I can fall through the earth, go far away where I can disappear.

Anger workshop could not have come at a more perfect time. Our group is moved to a larger room for this class led by a petite lady with tightly spiraled red curls holding a bucket of clay with all the colors of the rainbow. She draws on the board with a blue magic marker and explains that anger is normal, but we have to control it so it doesn't overtake us outwardly as rage or inwardly as depression. The dots connect for me. When I was younger and more of a perfectionist I was always depressed because I had so much anger I wasn't supposed to express. Later, when I could feel that I was full of anger, it finally bubbled over. I was seething with it.

The red-haired lady explains that it's important to realize why we're angry and let it out in a productive way before it turns to rage or depression, so we're going to throw the clumps of clay at a large vertical board across the room.

The exercise is not just about physically throwing the clay but also giving a voice to the anger. I'm interested but self-conscious. I know I'm angry, but I don't know if I can form my anger into words other than profanity. A few girls take their turns. The red-haired lady stands them about ten feet from the board, hands them chunks of clay, and repeats the beginning, which is always the same.

"I have a right to my anger," the redhead says.

"I have a right to my anger," a girl repeats and whips the clay. With a loud thud it hits the board.

"My anger is valid," says the redhead.

"My anger is valid," the girl repeats. Thud, like a brick hitting skin with an empty echo.

"I'm angry," she says.

"I'm angry." Thud.

"Who are you angry at?" asks the redhead

"I'm angry at God." Thud.

"Okay pretend you're talking to Him," says the redhead.

"God, I'm angry at You." Thud.

The girl's story begins to unravel as the redhead asks questions to keep the anger flowing. The clay smashes loudly and sticks in colored chunks where it hits the wall. The room is absolutely silent except for some of us who are crying as she hurls the colored chunks, as her voice gets soft and waivers, as she can barely continue on, as the redhead has to remind her to throw the clay and keep throwing and keep talking instead of breaking down. With each girl it's the same. They are left shaking, standing in front of us, breathing heavily as we clap for them and cry for them, and with them, in the fragile moment of sharing all of our deepest pain. How God has failed us, how our parents have failed us, how some of us have been abused or sexually exploited, how we resort to hurting ourselves because we all just want to be loved and accepted as we are.

I'm crying because if I met these people on the street I'd never be able to guess all the pain they hide. I'm crying also because I feel guilty. My life was nice, my parents were there, and they loved me. I was never abused. I was never unloved. How can I face the anger wall with nothing to say except that I want to be skinny? The guilt impales me. Sometimes I wish I'd had a horrible life so I'd have an excuse. How can I throw clay when I am angry and I have no real reason why? I feel like I'm failing this exercise. *I'm angry. Throw clay. Why? I'm angry because I'm angry. Throw clay. Why? Well, if I knew that, I probably wouldn't be as angry, now, would I? OK, I'll sit back down. Yeah, I wouldn't cry for that performance either. But if I don't figure out why I'm angry, I'll never get better.*

9

THE PEDESTAL OF GREATNESS

Meals suck, as usual. The dietician finally agrees to lower my milk consumption in exchange for upping my veggies and fat. She also informs me that I can't eat peanut butter and jelly for breakfast and lunch, even though I tell her it's what I'm going to do anyway when I leave this place, because it's what I like to eat. She's not amused. The food is solidifying into a concrete slug inside my intestines, and I'm bloated and constipated. I have a headache, and my side is beginning to hurt.

Now that I have the numbers to a phone card, I can call my dad, who thanks me for the coffee I sent him from the place where I work and asks me if I have a cold because I sound different. I'm covering the mouthpiece tightly with my palm until the second I speak, and then I cover it up again, so no small sound from the hospital can fill his mind with questions. I'm a liar, a big fat liar, and I vent my frustration during group therapy.

One of the girls tells me she had the same problem with her family, and she was shocked at how supportive they turned out to be. Another girl puts it differently: "If your best friend were in here instead of you, would you want to know?"

"Yes," I say, getting a new perspective with my answer.

She tells me how lying and hiding are not being honest with the real me. She says I'm also missing out on the support that I could be receiving from my family and friends, because they care about me. She gives me a little advice about setting boundaries and explains that I don't have to tell them every single thing. Instead, I could say something like I wasn't in a place of good health, so I've gone somewhere to recover. Or I could say I have an unhealthy relationship with food, and I'm here in the hospital so I can work on that. She tells me that I don't even have to say the words, "I have an eating disorder," because I can set the boundaries for myself and let people know only as much as I tell them, as much as I want to reveal.

The whole conversation is like an introduction to a foreign language. *Setting boundaries? What does that even mean?* How did they know that they could say such things and not reveal the scariest words, "I have an eating disorder." In bold letters I write *SET BOUNDARIES* on my list of things to research how to do.

What are the things they call boundaries? Until I got here, I thought I had the perfect family. We were so close and so tightly knit. I prided myself on that, but what if I'd been living in an illusion and what I thought was close was in fact claustrophobic and unnatural? Everyone seemed to know about boundaries but me. If my parents asked a question, we answered. We were expected to pour ourselves on the floor, so they could see everything and lovingly go through the pieces, like putting together a puzzle.

Everyone does the best they can with what they have. Most parents are lovingly motivated, and yet no person comes out of childhood unscathed. We all have gaps and little cracks that we have to fill by our own means, our own devices. It doesn't mean that our parents failed us. Sometimes they didn't have the tools to give us. Sometimes it's up to us to put forth the effort to acquire the knowledge we need to be happy and healthy.

Whether I was trying to be perfect to earn my parents' love or others' acceptance, I felt that if I could just do things a certain way, everything would be under control, and I would be okay. My parents put me on a pedestal that kept me always climbing to try to live up to their great faith in me. But it was too much. If it were true that I had the potential to be phenomenal, then I could accept nothing less—nothing less than amazing.

Whenever my brother and I didn't believe in ourselves, we were told how great we were. I know it was my parents' way of building us up, but it backfired. They held me in such high regard, I couldn't share with them anything less than my greatness. I was embarrassed by my negative feelings, by anything that wasn't me shining on the pedestal, so I fell silent and no one could hear all my derogatory self-talk but me.

People view willpower, self-control, and abstinence as power, but when someone like me, with an insatiable drive for perfection, seeks that power, it can jump back to devour the thing I was seeking in the first place. Freedom.

Is that what I hunger for?

10

SLAP IN THE FACE

My stomach is full from peanut butter and jelly and coffee with too much soymilk. I'm seasick from the sloshing.

"I'm Christen."

"Hi, Christen."

"Um, three affirmations. OK. I love my ass."

"Yes, you do."

"I can accept my body as is."

"Yes, you can."

"Um. I am a beautiful, healthy person."

"Yes, you are."

When we affirm each other, I can feel the pain through our smiles, as though we want so badly for these things to be true, as if by stating them we can make them so, as if by affirming them aloud the person will know them as truth. The real truth is we all see the beauty in each other that none of us see in ourselves. Inaccurate thoughts produce inaccurate feelings. My pants being tight immediately tells me I'm fat, which tells me I'm disgusting, gross, inadequate, and undisciplined, which leads to starving, binging, and purging or to compulsive exercise.

Why do a fat ass and thighs bother me so much? Why do I panic when I look down and see they've grown and stretched? Why is there constant pressure to maintain thinness? Why do I fail at constant vigilance? The disorder makes me feel isolated and depressed, and the little kid within me fights against the restrictions and the anxiety, because that kid doesn't want to be tortured anymore. The happy girl I used to be doesn't want to be forced to run, to throw up, to politely refuse food with a smile when she would trade half her soul to eat a cupcake in peace and not get fat.

When I look back at pictures of me when I was a little kid, I seem so happy. My pigtails are decorated with neon green scrunchies. My front baby tooth hangs down lower than the others. I wonder what I used to think about. I can't quite remember what it felt like to be her, to be free. Today, in the mirror, she looks back at me with huge hazel eyes as if she knows that something in me still fights for her, however small and however weak she is. She waits patiently for me to find my way back, so we can be happy again.

Sometimes Lillie appears as a posse of demons that torture me until I give in. They harass me until I agree with what they say and their voice becomes my voice and their thoughts become my thoughts. They say, "You are weak, fat, disgusting, worthless, ugly, fat, fat, fat, fat, fat, fat." *I am weak, fat, disgusting, worthless, ugly, fat, fat, fat.* I am exactly what I tell myself every second of every day. My subconscious repeats, without me even knowing, *I am fat. I am fat. I am unacceptable. I am disgusting.* It whispers, *You will never be free of me because I am you and you are me.*

It's been five full days, and I've been forced to keep everything down, which is getting a little easier in some ways but harder in others. Every day I examine the sides of my belly to judge the density of fat. Under my scrutiny my body expands. My subconscious screams that I'm out of control. They're making me eat too much too often. I can feel my fat cells grab at all the starches and load them straight onto my thighs like a game of Tetris. It's unnerving, and yet there is a small spark of morbid excitement: I'm keeping food in my stomach all the time. Isn't that a sign I'm getting better?

When visiting hours roll around, I know Leon will be here. I called my parents and they said that he would. My mom and dad told me that they were so proud and completely supportive of me being in the hospital and getting help.

I join one girl's conversation with her visitor and pretty soon we're talking about cookies. The visitor gives us the name of a good vegan cookie book, then stops and says, "Should we be talking about food?" I know it's an honest question, but I feel like punching her in the face. Just because we have eating disorders doesn't mean we can't talk about food. It reminds me how naïve the rest of the world is about us. It reminds me that I can't confide in anyone who doesn't have the same eating disorder, because the person will misunderstand and say stupid things. I can imagine myself at the visitor's house, sitting and eating while she watches me and wonders how I eat and what I'm thinking, as if I'm on display, as if I'm different and should be observed with a careful eye.

Getting up to use the bathroom is my excuse for not going back to the conversation.

The yellow phone that brings Leon's voice to me presses against my ear. He says he's going to come visit me tonight. I tell him to bring a big fat cake. He is not amused, even though I'm kidding. Well, half-kidding.

11

SEEKING VALIDATION

A scale estimates the mass of a body. It does not measure happiness or freedom.

Never have I been a numbers kind of person. Not in math, not in science, not in my eating disorder. I've never cared how much I actually weigh but instead how my clothes fit and how I feel inside my body. I happen to know the number of pounds I weighed when I was the most fat and depressed, when my body felt like it was loaded with sludge and overstuffed with poisons, because I was weighed at the hospital visit. I couldn't care less about the number, because I keep a pair of jeans in the back of my closet that I can pull up only three-fourths the length of my thighs. I use the jeans to evaluate myself, not a number.

What would I like to measure on my scale? What I hunger for is to be great, to feel like I'm good enough. I want happiness and freedom. I want to be strong, to be bold, to stand up for myself, to have my feelings voiced and validated, to be justified, to be understood. I want to love my body and stop killing it, to feel self-confident, *to live*. I need to feel real—no secrets, no pretending. I want to be myself and have myself be someone I love.

When I was a little girl, around age eight, I stood in the living room having expressed some sort of emotion, like fear or apprehension. My dad, who always saw me through the lens of my potential, pushed my feeling aside and tried to boost my self-esteem.

"Why are you afraid? Don't be afraid. You are so smart. You can do it," he said.

Rather than disappoint him, I bottled my feelings. *I'm too smart to be afraid. What great faith my dad has in me. I can't show him how weak I am.* I pushed the feeling aside, and didn't fully express what was true for me, because my feelings went invalidated.

I pretended I didn't feel sad. *Why should I feel sad when I've been blessed with so much?* Knowing I was blessed didn't stop me from feeling—sad, afraid, or angry at times—but I didn't want to be thought of as weak, so I pretended nothing bothered me. What I needed was someone to tell me, "It's OK to have these negative emotions. You can feel that, and it's OK." Or even better, "Why do you feel that?"

How does it affect me years later? I excel in cognition. I'm ultra-aware. I intellectualize all of my feelings. I live in my head and ignore my body, which is weak. Anything weak must go. That's why I hate myself now, because I've reduced myself to this animalistic creature that craves food, exercise, binging, and throwing up, like a nympho craves sex. I'm a slave. All day long Lillie's voice is in my head, and she will not shut up. All day long I have to fight not to lose control. All day long I'm physically present but a thousand miles away, because all I want is for people to leave, so I can be alone with my food and my toilet and the darkest part of me. I can't think of anything else, but even when I get what I want, the pleasure is fleeting and I want more and more and more. I'm another weak and worthless addict, and the result is always the same lie.

Before breakfast at the hospital I speed walk around the square of grass for fifteen minutes and wonder if I'm actually burning more than maybe five calories. Since high school I've known that it takes about a mile run to burn off a banana. Running is not even an option here, and they're making me eat a hell of a lot more than a banana. Sometimes I picture myself yelling really loudly directly into the dietician's face. Other times, when she hands my meal plan back for me to revise, I just shrug. It's all so exhausting. If they won't let me burn off anything, what's the point of adding calories on top of calories? I can see the justification in not eating at all. Too bad I also love food.

This afternoon we're told that we're going to a different part of the hospital to attend an Overeaters Anonymous meeting. The walk down the hallway past the gates fills me with dread. Most of us inpatients are what people would consider skinny. Why would they think it's a good idea to send us to a support group for people who are usually pretty large? Isn't that cruel?

We file into the room and take our seats as all the OA members watch. If I could hear people's thoughts, I know they'd be saying they hate us for being skinny. I keep thinking that we're cheaters, because they're just like us except they don't purge.

We don't accept the consequences for our disease. We don't let the food sit inside us so others can see it hanging off our frames. They must hate us. Some of them are quite large, but some appear normal and I wouldn't especially notice them walking down the street. I wouldn't even point them out as overweight. One of the women talks about how she ate a whole birthday cake in one sitting when bad memories of a childhood birthday resurfaced. Another talks about needing to attend meetings for the rest of his life. I watch as all the others nod in agreement. I sit there baffled, feeling guilty for being skinny even though I tell myself I'm fat. It must be hard, having to live the rest of their lives going to meetings to stay recovered. I feel sad for them. They're on a seesaw, and it's only a matter of time before something falls. There has to be another way to balance, because there's no way I can live the rest of my life resisting something as powerful as food. And I also can't spend the rest of my life giving in.

Sara has a dark sense of humor about this place. We sit at the same assigned table where we eat lunch and talk. Without her I could mistake this place for a boot camp. The others eat as fast as they can. *Just get through the meal. Just get through this meal. Just shoot me if this is going to be my life.* There has to be a way for my thoughts to eradicate any tie with food, with eating, with throwing up, with wanting to starve. I don't want to just get through life. I want to love it. I want to enjoy all my food and not think about whether it's making me fat or where the bathroom is.

Sara is a blast. When she first walked into the fish tank, I noticed her. She's blonde and looks like a Barbie. Naturally, I hated her immediately. But in spite of myself, once I started talking to her I realized we were a lot alike.

Formerly anorexic, now bulimic, both of us can turn our stomachs, and both of us are sarcastic. We love to share stories and joke about what we'd be eating if we weren't in prison. She's the only person who doesn't turn into a mute zombie when the meals come. And did I mention she's witty and kind and loves to laugh? In the mornings, we walk little laps around the grass square together and chat about things to see them from a comical perspective. Now that she's here, I can't imagine this deranged summer camp without her.

Today, in group therapy, a girl tells us that her husband has given up on her and says he's waiting for her to mess up. She says he's not supportive or caring or affectionate anymore. She sees the letter I received from Leon and tells me that she wrote two letters to her husband and asked him to please write back, but he hadn't. It hurts my heart, and at the same time it makes me feel so grateful for Leon's support and love.

I think about Leon. Why the hell doesn't he leave me? I think about how I should've decided not to get involved, not to let someone get attached to the best parts of me, because eventually the dark, putrid secrets are exposed, too. I can only lock Lillie in the closet for so long before she comes out to rip my life to shreds and dance in the confetti.

Leon is the main reason I'm not dead. When it comes right down to it, I'd throw my life away, but I won't throw his away, yet that's what I've been doing every day.

After making more than ten calls to Julie, I finally get her on the phone. My heart is beating in loud thuds as I tell her about how I want to be thin and how I binge on sweets and want to eat more and more. I leave out the purging part, because I'm uncomfortable being honest about it . . . because I think she won't want to be my friend if she really knows me. She seems concerned and worried. When I hang up the phone I feel some relief and a bit of guilt, because I can't come completely clean. I'm too afraid and ashamed of people seeing me for what I have become.

*

The yellow phone brings my dad too close for comfort, rubs up right against the raw part of me.

"How are you?"

"I had a good day. I talked a lot with Sara, and we had goal groups, and I told Julie the truth except about the purging part."

"Do you feel it's good for you to be in there?"

"What? Yeah. I've realized a lot of things, like how much high school messed me up, how uncomfortable I was all the time, how alone I felt all the time, like I never fit in."

"I don't know why you can't just let it go, because it all happened in the past."

I almost yell, "I didn't know it was still such a problem. It's like the eating disorder in the first place. You think that I can take some magic little pill and, poof, it's gone, or think hard enough and I can overcome it mentally."

"I believe the mind is stronger," he says.

"But dad, this is what I'm saying: it's a disease, a disorder. An eating disorder is not something I can wish away. I can't take some fucking magic pill, or else I'd have done that already."

"It's classified as a disease?"

What I want is for you to understand, to validate what I've unearthed about my childhood, how I felt my feelings weren't validated. Instead, my feelings bounce off of you, and you put your own in their place. "The point is, Dad, that I feel guilty and weak when you think it's something I can just get over. I feel guilty and weak, like it's my fault, like I'm too weak to just get over it."

"I'm not saying that at all."

"But that's how I feel, Dad. That's how I feel." *There he goes again, devaluing my feelings. It's a feeling.* "You're not listening to me," I say. "You're not hearing what I'm saying."

"How can you say that? I always listen to every word you say."

Give up, my mind says. *Just give up, stay silent, don't argue. I realize that you saw all my pain, Dad. You felt it all with me. Your heart hurt for me so deeply, but you couldn't change that I was dwindling away, that I would run during my lunch breaks, that I always felt alone. You didn't know the details, but you knew you couldn't save me. And I wanted so much to be like you. I wanted to be strong and in-your-face, so on the outside I was such a great pretender, but on the inside, I shriveled.*

I have no balance. I have no equanimity, just an emptied out feeling wanting to be filled with validation.

My dad interrupts the silence. "Think about what I said. Don't worry about hurting my feelings. If you think it would be better not to talk to us while you're there, if it hinders your progress. Think about it."

You are my biggest supporter and greatest nemesis. "I will," I say. "Love you."

"Love you, too."

I blow a mouthy kiss and click the yellow phone receiver back down on its hook, my brain swimming in all the words I never say. I leave them smoldering in the hallway.

I go back to my room and write a scathing letter that I will never send.

I am empty now.

Me.

12

DON'T LET THE SHRINKS TWIST YOUR HEAD

I sleep like a fiend—deep, and dark, and dreamy with pictures swirling in my head like cream in coffee.

Later, my feet press into the carpet as I fidget in the chair in the tiny little room with my therapist, Margaret. Reading to her my letter about the phone call with my dad makes me nervous, because I don't express to others how I feel, and I don't read aloud to people what I write.

"How does that make you feel?" she asks when I'm silent.

I feel sadness, because I never believed all the good things about myself. I idolized my dad and wanted his in-your-face strength, because I despise weakness.

"Could you read the letter you wrote, about your father, to him?" She leans forward towards me as a show of support.

Overcome with emotion, I tell her absolutely not, because he would take it personally. He doesn't get it. He gets all hurt and upset, as though I'm telling him he was a horrible father, when in no way was that the case. He would stay up all night and take it all wrong and blow it out of proportion. The more I picture him, I find I'm crying in her office as she offers the support she anticipated I would need. I cry because I feel so awful. I know that both of my parents did everything out of love for my brother and me. My dad did everything from love, and he always tried to protect me and save me from pain, but he hurt *with* me. He said he wished he could take my place, but I didn't want to cause him any pain or hurt, so I kept everything inside to minimize my effect on those who loved me.

Margaret looks perturbed. "When you don't express emotions because of your parents' reaction to them, that's just another way of not validating your feelings." She goes on to explain that I was taught or trained not to express emotion, and to fear its expression, because of the uncomfortable reactions I got in return.

The discomfort led me to bottle my feelings and tell myself, *Whatever. It doesn't matter. It shouldn't matter.*

Half of my energy is spent thinking, the other half is spent trying to hold back tears so she won't witness my fragility. "No," is my immediate and almost forceful reply. I soften the edge a bit and continue, "No, because they would feel like I'm going behind their backs. I know for sure that my dad would tell you something like 'I appreciate you talking with Christen, and that's great she's learning, if it helps her, but I know my daughter and love her, and who are you to tell me . . .' et cetera, et cetera."

My voice trails off as I remember clearly what he said to me when I described the program at the hospital. I hear his voice as though it's been recorded and played back in my head: "Don't let the shrinks twist your head." I cringed on the inside.

We end up talking about what strength means to me. Margaret describes bridging the gap between the adult me and the young girl who held the green plastic lunchbox, when, in a moment of courage, she went to the cafeteria. Margaret gestures like she's holding a lunch box in front of her, and I start crying again.

Her eyes tear and she turns her lips down in an empathetic nod. "You're still in touch with that girl in high school, and you're going to have to find a way to bridge the gap between her and who you are now."

"How?" I almost whisper. When I feel such devastating sadness for her, for the naïve girl holding the lunchbox full of terrified hope, for who I used to be?

"We bridge the gap by facing our emotions, not stuffing them down with food, or starving them away, or throwing them up."

"Yeah, but it's scary," I say.

She breathes out slowly and looks me in the eyes like a mother would. "It can't be worse than what you're doing to yourself."

A huge breath makes its way into my lungs as though I'm inhaling her words. I let it out, heavy and thick, and nod because my mouth feels like it's stuffed full of dry bread, and even if I could speak, the words would come out jumbled in fragments like sawdust.

13

POISONING MY SPIRIT WITH FOOD

When I'm preoccupied with battling the urge to throw up my food, the days feel excruciatingly long. Yesterday, I was physically tired and could tell that my food was digesting at a sluggish snail's pace. I'm constipated and feeling heavy and tight. Eating breakfast pushes me over the edge. The first bite nauseates me like I'm forcefully stuffing food into a body that's already hoarding food, bloated, lazy, sick, and poisoned.

"Margaret, eating this much is unhealthy. I'm never hungry when I eat here. How is that healthy?"

"What do health and healthy mean to you?" she asks.

"Look. I feel like when I overeat I'm just stuffing food on top of more undigested food, and when I'm full all day long my body doesn't have time to rest. I equate that with sickness."

"How does this belief system hinder your recovery?" she says.

"In about every way," I say. "It makes it hard to deal with my body image and food as related to my eating disorder. I know my beliefs. I've read about a lot of so-called strange, unorthodox ways of eating, and I believe in them, not just because I want to be skinny but because I believe in them."

"Give me an example," she says.

"Like fasting. Like the fact that most of what people eat is not what the body is designed to process. The ideal way to eat is raw. But people keep trying to tell me I have these belief systems because of the eating disorder, and

I want to punch them in their fucking faces when they say that."

"But you do have an eating disorder."

"I know," I sigh. "It's a catch-22. I know at the same time that what I'm doing to my body is not right either. I know that the anorexia and bulimia are not healthy, but I can't stop, even though I know the right way."

"So what's holding you back from giving up the eating disorder?"

"I know what I should do. I just feel like it controls me. It comes down to purity of body, purity of spirit. It's a battle between spirituality, food, and my eating disorder. I never started off wanting to be skinny as my goal. I started off wanting to be healthy and pure."

"Yes, that's a tricky situation. You're walking a fine line because you have an eating disorder."

When I leave her office and walk down the florescent-lighted hallway back to the eating disorders unit, I can't help but wonder how I'll end this war between my eternal soul and the physical body that's supposed to be my temple.

In the stall in the bathroom I'm crying from the frustration of being forced to eat things I feel are bad for me. The nutritionist actually suggested I eat oatmeal or pancakes for breakfast, which makes me want to throw my pencil in her stupid eyeball. She knows full well I believe they clog my intestines. I redo the menu and go to the bathroom and cry with the knot in my throat and my anxiety rising. I check my emotions as I sit there staring down at my feet and realize that I'm angry, frustrated, and conflicted about food. At the deep dark bottom, I'm afraid.

Oatmeal. Just the word pierces me with anxiety. Oatmeal is binding, like sludge, in my intestines. I'm terrified my body will shut down like it did before and no doctors will be able to find anything wrong, just like before, and they'll tell me again that it's all in my head. Even more than the side pain, I'm scared of the anger that comes with it, the rage and the hopeless depression. No one knows how dark a space I will go to. I can see them telling me that it's just a phase—that I feel this way because I have an eating disorder. This isn't normal. I know it's not, but no one will listen to me. Once again I'll be alone—me and the body I hate that's now starting to punish me back. All of this explodes with just one little word: oatmeal.

14

THE SHADE UNDER THE TREE

With nothing to do on Saturday, I feel bored. My goal is to be positive all day. Starting now. There's no set schedule other than meals, so I take my time laying out a blanket on the grass under the shade of a tree.

Leon and Julie come to see me, because the visiting hours are longer on the weekends. They arrive together, so I show them my collage, and we sit inside and play Trouble, the little board game with the plastic bubble in the center. We're all trying to pretend we're in Julie's living room instead of at the eating disorder hospital. Leon gets a phone call, so he goes out into the courtyard and paces little circles around a tree. Julie and I sit there in an awkward silence.

"I brought some nail polish, so I can paint your nails if you want," she offers.

This makes me happy. "Yes. I'd love that."

She reaches into her purse and pulls out a plastic bag containing a purple polish. "What's it like to be in here?"

"It's sort of like camp in a weird, prison style. The food sucks. We eat three meals and two snacks, whether we want to or not, and we pretty much live in this fish tank room all day, so it's strange. Everything is controlled, and that's probably the part I hate the most. But on the good side, I like Ellie and Sara. We've become friends." I point to Ellie, just waking up from her nap, wrapped in her blue blanket that looks like a cocoon, and Sara sitting cross-legged with all her papers scattered around her as she frantically juggles her cigarette from hand to hand like a hot potato.

"Has this been going on since high school?" she asks.

"What do you mean?"

"Well… everyone knew you were anorexic then," she says.

This catches me off guard, and I'm silent for a few seconds as she passes the brush over my nails that now glitter a deep purple. *Everyone knew? I thought I hid it so well.* Only one girl on my basketball team ever confronted me about it. I remember sleeping over at Julie's house, and she asked me if I was okay. I told her I was and ended the conversation.

"Everyone knew?"

She looks up, a little embarrassed, "Well, yeah, you were pretty skinny. It was kind of obvious."

"Huh." I stare back down at my nails.

Leon sits back down and rattles off something about his parents. I feel boring and embarrassed that I can't leave or actually do anything with them but sit. We discuss how, when I get out, we can have a barbeque and do some Jacuzzi time at Julie's house. After a while we've run out of plans for our pretend barbeque, so we have our goodbyes, and I watch them walk through the gate I cannot pass.

That night, Ellie and I curl up on the couch in her blue cocoon blanket and watch half of *White Oleander* together. A few days ago I put in a request to move to Ellie and Sara's room, because it has an unoccupied bed. For now, we've been spending late hours in the common spaces so we can hang out together longer.

"Are they finally going to let you move into our room?" Ellie asks, yawning.

"Oh, yeah, I forgot. Sorry. They said I could move tomorrow morning. It only took them three days to get back to me."

"Yay! I'm excited. Sara decorated it this afternoon and put up some of the collages so the room looks more homey." She smiles, and it warms me from the inside. She never used to talk to anyone, and now she talks to me.

15

IF YOU CAN'T BE HONEST

"If you can't be honest, you won't recover," says one of the girls this morning at breakfast while I'm trying to force oatmeal down my throat against an almost immediate gag reflex. In the bathroom I sit on the toilet for ten minutes trying to convince myself not to throw up and wishing the nutritionist would miss a few steps and tumble head-first down the stairs for forcing me to eat things my body cannot handle.

Today, a few of us are approved for an outing to Starbucks. We walk in a small group with the leader, Rachel, who is our babysitter for the day. Ellie, Sara, and I walk together on the sidewalk and point out cool-looking trees or beautiful flowers and talk about our dream houses. As we enter the parking lot of Starbucks I'm slightly afraid of seeing other people, especially since we're noticeable in a group with an obvious caretaker figure. I suddenly realize we're all wearing hospital bracelets—something that has become so normal to me I don't think about it. Now, in the normal world again, I feel the white plastic around my wrist and wish I were invisible. I tell myself I'm strong. I tell myself I don't care what other people think. I tell myself they won't notice. We order coffee, and I can taste my anxiety like thick whipped cream in my mouth—solid and fatty and blocking my throat. Everyone is watching us, or at least it feels that way to me. I have to go outside where I can breathe.

Rachel, our babysitter, has pulled a couple of tables together and some chairs.

"I hate that everyone is watching us," I tell her.

"Yeah, but just don't think about it."

"This latte tastes amazing," I say, taking a thankful sip even though I'm full from lunch.

She looks at me. Her key card is hanging from a lanyard around her neck. "It gets easier," she says. "I promise."

My eyes avert, so I won't break down crying right there. Sara had told me that she was pretty sure some of our babysitters were previous patients, but they wouldn't tell us for sure. To know that Rachel honestly knows what I'm going through makes me feel like I'm seen. Not as someone in the eating disorders unit of the hospital, but seen as a real person by someone who isn't trying to analyze me or make it better. If they could tell the truth, I feel like our babysitters would say, "I see you and I acknowledge and respect your struggle to get better."

Ellie walks up and silently drops a newspaper on the table.

Sara pulls a chair out next to me, sits down, and takes a sip of her coffee. "That was kind of uncomfortable," she says and tells me that inside some mother and daughter were looking at Ellie and Sara and whispering and giggling. She holds up her bracelet arm. "I wish I could rip this off. I'm pissed I didn't think to bring my sweatshirt."

I glance over at Ellie who's scanning the newspaper and seems to have shut out the whole table.

"Did you say anything to them?" I ask Sara.

"No," she laughs. "What am I supposed to say?"

"I don't know," I say, "something like 'what the hell is so funny?'" Sara shrugs and takes another sip of her coffee. I know she's too nice to say anything like that.

"Maybe they weren't even talking about you," Rachel says.

Stop being naïve, I think. Of course they were laughing about us, but what I can't figure out is why?

*

That night, Ellie and I make a huge birthday card for one of the outpatient girls. Ellie glues some stars we cut out onto the construction paper as I read her my journal entry about the trip to Starbucks. She gets quiet.

"What's wrong? Are you okay?" I ask.

She looks up at me with a little smile. "It's just that you wrote about me in your journal."

"Um, yeah, you were a part of my day." I wonder if this is not OK in some way.

"No, I mean when I heard you read, it made me happy because I knew that when I die, you will have remembered me."

I don't know what to say to this, to the fear that we will all die and our lives will have been lived unnoticed. That we make no impact on the world or other people. That all we do is take up space in a body, a life that could have been fuller and happier. When she dies she hopes she'll be remembered. Isn't that what we all want, to live a happy life and leave an imprint on the world, a lasting legacy that proves we didn't exist in vain, that proves we matter, that we're worth it?

16

HOW GRAY IS A SAFE COLOR

Just when I may be starting to like the hospital, the nutritionist increases all my food rations. I'm pissed and cry hateful tears. I'm terrified because my side pain has returned, and now they want to give me more food. Do they not listen to what I'm saying? Why are they trying to stuff me like a pig? After lunch, I go back to my room and cry some more because I feel fat and gross and poisoned.

Jackie, comes in specifically to tell me that I am not allowed to have prunes because of the eating disorder's tendencies.

I'm trying not to cry. "But I need them to take a shit, because if I can't go, my side will hurt even more. I can't go back to that place again."

She gives a snide little smile, very masculine. "Well, if you stop going to the bathroom, I'll know that you're telling the truth."

As she walks away I picture throwing my journal like a boomerang. I watch as it snips her head off her body. What a bitch. I am not making this up.

In art class the teacher has us coloring mandalas, and I'm coloring and crying everywhere. Ellie and Sara look at me and nod. They know there's nothing they can do. None of us has power here. "Sorry, babe," Sara says and doesn't take it personally when all I do is nod back. Ellie moves her crayons a little closer to me so I can share all her colors.

They're playing music as we shade the mandala patterns. The music makes me view myself as a child again, when I was happy. I can see myself in the pictures my parents have in their old photo albums. There is one in particular of a day at the zoo. The sun is streaking across the page like a flashlight, and I'm standing on the grass with my hands reaching up in the air as if I'm trying to gather the light from the sky.

That seems like a whole lifetime ago. Where did that little girl go? Finally, I leave art therapy. The music is just too much. I sit on my bed and cry and draw circles with the red pen I took. Does this disease ever end? I'm such a smart girl. Why can't I just stop the thoughts and feelings? Why can't I look at food like a normal person? Normal people don't cry when their prunes are taken away. Normal people don't have people taking away their prunes in the first place.

17

THE SEDUCTION

Lillie,

You came like a shadowed stranger with a hint of oleander scent. You filled the empty spaces, the voids where I had no words. You were my salvation when my world teetered. You said it would be easy. You said that I was brilliant to have discovered a way to not get fat. You said you would protect me, that it would be all right. I opened the door, invited you in, soft and shy the hope of the dream behind a black overcoat slipping puddles off the hanger to the floor. Your lips are deep purple and they're on mine and mine on yours, your breath in my mouth, our fingers lock your hips, my hips, your hands, my hands, darkness, darkness, my belly, your hands, my hands, whisper, whisper. You lied.

Where do you end? Where do I begin?

Dear Body, my temple, my enemy, my best friend,

When I was little we used to be best friends. We would laugh, build dams, swim at the pool, fly kites at the park, and ride bikes to get Fudgesicles. We'd laugh as the sun burned us brown and lie exhausted reading Nancy Drew. Then one day I decided you were not good enough for me, and I decided to make you my slave.

I destroyed you with a vengeance—beat you down until you were what I wanted you to be. I took away your intellect and forced you to run instead of making friends, forced you to eat only what I told you was okay. I'm sorry for breaking your heart every time I looked in the mirror and hated what I saw in you.

Nearly every day, I promised to stop hurting you and broke those promises minutes later. Even though I poisoned, restrained, and belittled you daily, you continued to function and live. Thank you for fighting for me so I could fall in love with Leon and he could see your beauty, because I never did.

I am truly sorry, and I will work hard to be better for us so we can be free and happy.

Love,

Christen Z.

18

TREMENDOUS GUILT

Rumor has it there may be a genetic link to eating disorders, which means absolutely nothing, except that we who have them are born with a slight tendency in that direction.

In school, I was the weird kid who brought corn and peas in Tupperware with my lunch. My mom and I baked cookies and brownies together because, like me, she has a sweet tooth. My brother and I were her best friends, but as we grew older she still saw us as little kids. She would say, "Oh, do you think it's a good idea to drive all the way out there by yourself?" She instilled fear in us so we'd stay childlike and not grow up and do things on our own. She wanted to be our best friend. She didn't like being alone.

She told me all she ever wanted was for me to be happy. I think she feared me hating her, and that's why she never came straight out and talked to me about my eating disorder. She avoided the issue, pretended it wasn't a pink elephant. Maybe she thought if I was pretending to be happy, I was. I think she had no idea what to do. Maybe she was, in her own way, trying to heal me by taking me to food, like cattle to a water hole, and making sure I ate.

I was depressed, so she tried to make me happy by being my companion. My mom took me on many lunch dates. My silence made her uncomfortable, so she spent most of the time talking at me. She used her voice to try to fill the void between us.

I didn't deserve love. I didn't deserve her efforts to make me happy with the restaurant outings, spending time together, and conversation. I was a bad person. I was moody. I'd ruin family outings.

Guilt comes in painful jolts to my head and my heart. My father. My mother.

Dear Mom,

I love you. You were the best mom I ever could have asked for. You were always there for me to help my mind grow. You read to me and told me stories to spur my imagination. You kept me creative, dying t-shirts, doing Paint 'N' Swirl, finger-painting, Legos, puzzles, and Play-Doh. You gave us puppet shows when we had blackouts, and you'd chase us around the house with the vacuum and give us blanket rides across the living room floor. You'd take us to the beach for picnics and up to the pool. You let me try out every available sport and class to see what I liked. You helped us with our homework and spent all your waking time with us.

It is because of you sparking my brain that I am creative. You unselfishly cared and gave of yourself and showed me compassion and loving kindness. You were a steady foundation from which I grew.

It must have been so sad for you to give me such inspiration as a child and then see my happiness shrivel but not be able to control it. You couldn't fix it and make it better. I'm sorry for letting this disorder take away precious moments of our relationship. I'm sorry for throwing up food you took your love and time to buy and bring to me. I'm so sorry for being mean and hateful when all you were doing was trying to help me, when you were afraid and I treated you poorly or shut you out.

I would like to tell you how deeply I appreciate how you've always been there for me, how you don't judge me, and how you let me be myself.

I would like to be free from this eating disorder, so I can spend time with you and you can spend time with the real me, the core that you instilled, and all the fun new things I can bring to the table. I'd like to start a fresh page and erase all the past, all the guilt I felt about my eating disorder and how it separated me from you. I love you, Mom.

Love,

Your daughter, Christen

19

EMBRACING THE DARKNESS

I wish God gave out do-overs, so I could go back and not choose this path, not pigeonhole myself into this disease and waste my potential. If I could have a do-over, I'd go back to when I was a kid, because when I was little, God was always there for me. I had a strong sense that I was His child, that He listened to my prayers, and that He did in fact answer all of my requests.

Then, at age fifteen, when I met Lillie, everything I believed about God was tested. Food and God became intertwined. If I have enough faith, God should be able to heal me, right? Since He hasn't, that must mean I'm a bad person. I must be doing something wrong. My prayers are frantic and begging. *No, God. I can do better this time. Give me one more chance. I'll prove I'm not a failure. I know I should have no other gods before You.* But I do. Food is my idol, the toilet is my porcelain god, the skinny girls in the magazines are my golden images.

Food in the hospital is becoming a problem lately. All the food is beginning to make my side hurt. It's reminding me of how sick I was when I studied abroad in Germany, when I believed God had left me.

When my box of clothes arrived to my host family's house, I remember feeling stupid for thinking I could eat gelato, and laugh, and pretend to be normal. When I began to binge again the side pain started and I sunk into depression. I'd sit in the shower in the basement with all the lights off. It was ice cold and pitch black as the water ran over me. I once whispered, "Satan, are you in here?" For a few seconds I waited and listened to the water slam against my body and wash down the drain.

The doctors in Germany thought maybe my kidney had failed, but the test results were normal. Every time I visited a different doctor, the school translator had to accompany me. After being told a few times that there was nothing wrong with me, I felt guilty for taking up her time.

I began to drink for the first time in my life. I stayed out all night long, because I no longer gave a fuck. I threw up most of my meals, which was the only way I could relieve the pressure in my side. I began to take laxatives in large quantities. I didn't want to feel anything anymore. I wanted to be pleasantly numb and die peacefully.

I embraced the darkness, called it my own, made it my friend, and pulled it behind me quietly like a shadow.

20

A GOOD BITCH-SLAPPING

Lately, the shadow is creeping back. The nurse hands me my salad. Its toppings are larger than restaurant size, and it takes me an hour to finish eating it. The pain in my side comes back like a fist. I go to the bathroom to cry. Maybe because I feel better being close to the toilet, so if I want to throw up I can. I haven't yet.

Sara, my sole talking companion during meals, is waiting to tell me that Jackie is completely ignoring Sara's symptoms. Over the last week, Sara has been swelling. She's told them that the food they're making her eat has too much salt for her body to handle. They don't seem to care, and the diuretics are doing nothing but making her dizzy. At lunch today, her vision was blurred. We walk around the hallways just to move, and I'm burping up the air in my stomach so it will take away some of the full feeling and I won't want to throw up as much. "Sorry," I say. "My dad used to get pissed when I did this."

She smiles and shakes her head. "You're burping, and I'm going blind."

We laugh halfheartedly because we know it's not funny.

"So are they going to do anything for you? Obviously, you're not getting any less swollen."

"I talked to a different therapist today who validated my frustration with Jackie and actually acknowledged my symptoms were not normal."

"You think?" I add sarcastically.

She scuffs her fuzzy boots on the floor as we turn around and backtrack under the florescent lights.

"I think Jackie hates women and is especially jealous of pretty, intelligent ones."

"Yeah, that's probably why she's a bitch to me and completely ignores you." I like how Sara has personally pulled me aside to talk to. It makes me feel validated as a friend, like I'm special, like I belong.

"You know I hate this word," she says, "but she's kind of a cunt."

"Yeah, I don't think I ever say that word, but I agree . . . she's a big cunt. Let's call it something different."

"Like a cnook?" Sara looks hopeful.

"Yes. I say, let's shorten it to nook. The nook Nazi. I like that."

Sara laughs. "The nook Nazi. Let's go tell Ellie."

*

A new inpatient arrives. My frustration builds as I observe the flaws in their system. Her pain medication had worn off. They wouldn't give her another dose, because they hadn't approved it yet, so she sat in a chair, writhing in pain. She couldn't eat her snack because she was so nauseated. On top of that they almost refused to give her any Crystal Light, because it wasn't on her menu. We all stood up for her and told them the situation was ridiculous, so she's now sipping orange Crystal Light out of a paper cup. One point for the hospital girls. They told us they made the exception only because she's sick.

"She's sick because she needs her pain medication," I say, as though it's clear the nurses are morons. I get the eye, which means to shut up. "And what about Sara?" I ask.

"What exactly do you mean?" the nurse says.

"Well, for starters, she's swollen up like a marshmallow and has severe pitting edema in her legs, and no one is telling her what's going on."

Our babysitter for the day shifts her pen to the other hand. "If it's a big deal, Sara should be asking, not you."

"She did ask, many times, and no one's getting back to her."

"Sara is not your responsibility," she says.

Yes, she is, because I'm the one who is watching her get dizzy. I watched her involuntarily throw up today, because her equilibrium is off. I'm the one poking her legs at night and trying to massage the swelling down because no one is telling her anything. "This place sucks," I say, getting up.

"Where are you going?" she asks.

"To the bathroom."

"You have to wait until everyone has eaten their snack."

"But I have to pee," I say. She looks up at me like I'm not worth talking to anymore. I glare at the walls and turn my chair around, so I can't see any part of her, not even in my peripheral vision.

*

Ellie curls her hands into her black sweatshirt when she says she never lets God into her sad place. She says she won't allow herself to believe that God loves her because she won't allow His love into her sad place of self-hatred.

I know that God wants me to be healthy, but maybe I'm the one that interprets healthy equals thin. Is that my misconception? I don't think so. If you are clean and pure, the body is naturally thinner. I've never seen a fat raw foodist. The body is made up of the atoms of what we eat. If I didn't have an eating disorder, this whole belief system would make me weirdly health-conscious, but because I do have the disorder everyone blames my strange beliefs on the disorder. "Oh, she doesn't eat cheese because she's afraid of getting fat." *No, stupid. I don't eat cheese because it's a mucus-forming blob that will clog my intestines.*

I believe the hospital is poisoning us with massive quantities of dead food that the body can never use. This explains why my system has begun to clog and shut down again and my side is once again in pain. My body is begging me to stop eating. I'm scared of that powerless place where this pain takes me. Food no longer makes me happy. It disgusts me.

21

LONELINESS IS A BIG PART OF THE DISEASE

In my dreams I scream at a faceless stranger, "I've tried eating less, eating more, taking fiber, eating fruit, exercising, massaging my belly, walking, praying, eating prunes, drinking prune juice, taking colon cleanser, fasting, drinking water, drinking alcohol, taking massive amounts of laxatives, and finally throwing up every meal because it was the only way to stop the pain. If you can tell me what I haven't tried, please, be my guest. I would love for you to enlighten me."

The voice in my dreams whispers, "You haven't tried giving up the fear."

*

I wake from deep sleep feeling powerless. My stomach hurts. My side hurts. I feel like a bag of shit. Brush teeth, wash face, take shower. What's the point?

Back in our room, Ellie has folded all my underwear and shirts into little piles. How cute. The group is coloring mandalas in the fish tank room. I lean over to Sara and the other girl sitting at our table and whisper, "Hey, if the hospital won't give me prunes, I'm going to have Leon sneak me in some anti-constipation pills that I have left over from Germany."

"He agreed to that?" Today is the other girl's last day, because her insurance refuses to pay for more treatment, even though she throws up blood.

"He doesn't want to, but I begged him. They aren't listening to me, and if I refuse food that means I'm not compliant and have to drink shakes, and that means I won't be able to go on any outings, which is my only time away from this place."

"I completely understand," Sara says, holding up her colored mandala for us to see. "I'd do the exact same thing."

"Nice, I like the pink," I say. "Hey, Sara, the nook Nazi stole this book I was reading on eating disorders and put it with the contraband, but I was using it to write about my family."

"You want me to steal it back for you?"

"Well, I was just going to ask if you'd seen it, but, yeah, can you get it for me? It would help me with my writing."

"Consider it done," she says and smiles.

Later that night she slides into our room, where Ellie and I are silently collaging. She drops the book face up on the bed.

"I owe you one." I say.

22

THE JILTED LOVER SYNDROME

Growing up, I idolized my father. I would eat the same breakfasts—huge pieces of sourdough toast with orange cheese melting off the edges, or bagels and cream cheese. I'd wear his watch, which was almost the size of my palm. I slept with a long-sleeved t-shirt that smelled like him. He confided in me because I was smart, and I was a good listener. Although we didn't have a surplus of money, we didn't lack. My dad would wheel and deal to get us through the tough times.

I was the family therapist. Sensitive to others' feelings and adept at seeing all sides of a situation, I mediated. I was asked to talk to my brother when he got in trouble at school. "He'll listen to you."

My mom was nonconfrontational and overly kind. My dad was confrontational and brutally honest. If I didn't want to answer any question he asked, he took it as a personal rejection.

I often wanted to yell, "It's my life. It's *my* life!"

My family had no boundaries. I let family into all personal areas of my life without having any secrets, without holding anything that was just mine. If I did keep anything to myself, it was soon found out, and the interrogation would start and continue until I finally explained. I wanted a secret world. I wanted secrets that were all mine.

Even today, my father wants to know a lot. Only now that I'm married does he see me as somewhat out of the nest. Leon can fill his shoes by watching over me. If he didn't like Leon, he would make it difficult for me to be with him. His disapproving stares and little comments would come between Leon and me, like a wall, because I've always idolized my dad and sought his approval.

I thought I was the one who had fought so hard to be close to him, but when I began to pry myself away, he fought harder to hold on. I pushed and twisted and punched and bit and broke free running, but he grabbed a thread of my sweater and didn't let go.

23

THIS DISEASE

Before breakfast I give Ellie the collage I made for her with real colored leaves glued to construction paper sprinkled all over with silver and gold glitter. My stomach hurts, and they won't give me anything to help the bloating because they think I'm making it up. Could they be right? What if my side pain is a psychosomatic figment of my imagination? Or is it one of Lillie's dirty tricks?

Ellie is curled into her black hoodie as we sit outside on the sidewalk next to the little green square of lawn. Her long, blonde, straight hair falls loose at the edges of the hood and blows quietly in the breeze. The concrete is cold under my hands, and I can feel it through my jeans. "I am pissed at God," I tell her. "I mean, I'm making a huge, honest effort to get better, and I feel like I'm being punished again with this side pain, just like when I tried to get better in Germany."

She looks at me with her blank blue stare. "Yeah. No one believed me for over a year when I was super tired all the time, until finally I was diagnosed with fibromyalgia. Up until then everyone just thought I was making it up."

"Everyone's giving me the runaround. I have three of the anti-constipation pills from Germany, but I don't want to take them. They're just insurance."

She shrugs and scans the yard. "I would have taken them already. They obviously don't care."

"Yeah. I'm fucking pissed at how people think we don't know anything because we have eating disorders, but actually, we probably know our bodies so much better than any normal person ever will."

She pulls the cuffs of her sweatshirt over her fingers. "Do you think there's ever a better?"

My sigh is long and hollow and filled with all the words I don't know how to say. "I guess I have to hope there is, right? Otherwise what's the alternative? I guess anything is better than where I was."

She looks right at me. "I was happier," she says. "I only agreed to come here because my mom begged and cried."

"Wait," I say. "You didn't check yourself in?"

"Well, I guess I did, but not for the intention of getting better. Just to make my mom happy."

I want to hug her, but I don't. I want to make all the sadness pour out of her like water into the grass. I want to tell her that her life will be happy again, that everything will be OK. But I'm not even sure I can promise myself. I checked myself into the hospital with a flicker of hope that this would all, one day, turn out to be a sort of horrible nightmare. I want to put my arm around her, but I don't, so I just love her in silence—love her and myself at the same time.

24

YELLOW PHONES

There are only two phones we can use here. Both are neon yellow, situated in the middle of the hallway, and smack dab next to each other. This ensures that we have zero privacy. When two people are on the phones at the same time, one person is always having a more dramatic or painful conversation, and when that person is the other girl, it's hard for me to pay attention to my own conversation.

Ellie's on the phone next to me tonight. Leon's voice streams into my ear, but I'm distracted by Ellie crying on the phone next to me. She's already made a commitment to eat, she says, but it doesn't make everything go away. She must be talking to her mom. I tell Leon I'll call him later.

When she comes back into the room again she's silent and pulls a chair out at our table. "Do you need a hug?" I ask her quietly.

She shakes her head, "No. I'll be okay." We sit for a while. "My mom wasn't excited about me coming home," she finally says, looking up at me with her pale blue eyes.

"What do you mean, 'not excited'?"

Her hand curls around her sweater softly, like she's catching an orb of lint. "Well, I was supposed to go home pretty soon, until my therapist talked to my mom. Now my mom is convinced that I shouldn't come home until I get to a certain weight, so my brain can function normally."

"I think your brain's all right."

"Great. That makes two of us, and that won't get me home." A pained expression comes over her face. "I just don't get it. I've been eating everything I'm supposed to, and gaining weight, and I don't want to stay here anymore. I've done everything they've told me to."

There's nothing I can say, because I know it's true. She was here before I came and will be here after I leave, because she's the more difficult case, because she's too skinny, because they think her brain is not getting enough nutrition.

"It's just not fair . . . When I was taking my fibromyalgia medicine it made me sick and I lost weight and my intestines were all messed up and I felt like crap all the time and my family had this horrible ten-hour-long intervention, which was them just belittling me the whole time until finally I agreed to go to the hospital."

"You mean here?" I ask.

"No," she says, "the hospital I went to before. It was just to run all these tests. I ended up trying to gain weight, and I did, but then I was also restricting but didn't think I was. It was just so confusing. I didn't know if I was anorexic or not. I thought anorexic was not eating at all, but I was eating 300 calories a day."

"Um, dear, that's anorexic. I was anorexic eating 1000 calories a day."

She looks at me, perturbed, then fishes in her journal and pulls out a picture of her on vacation with her mom. She holds it up. They're smiling and pretty. I'm confused about when it was taken. "It was my birthday, so I ate cake and food and just didn't care—for about four days— and then when I went back home, I tried on a pair of my jeans, and I couldn't get them over my hips, and I freaked out. And thus began my descent into happiness."

The words linger there in the air for a moment, *my descent into happiness.*

"Into the hospital," I say, correcting her, but she shakes her head.

"My food, or lack of food, was a pride thing. It was like me saying to everyone, 'See? I don't need anything. I don't need my family. I'm sick of taking care of things. I'm even sick of food.' I was filled with pride when I didn't eat for a few days, and I had this huge sense of accomplishment."

"But were you actually happy, or did you miss eating?" I ask.

She leans back in her chair with a faraway look, "It was my thing. It made me happy, and all I wanted was for my mom to be happy that I was happy. I just wanted to die, fall asleep on the beach, and feel the warm sun. That little happiness I'd felt for that short time would be better than living and feeling the way I was before."

My breath is locked in my chest. Being from Hawai'i, I can picture this image so clearly—how she could smile, closing her eyes as the white light shines through the lids, how the sun would warm her whole body from above and the sand would be hot below, and how she could just fall asleep finally happy. I did the same thing when I was anorexic. I lay on the beach, closed my eyes, zoned out, and pictured myself miles away, somewhere where I was happy.

Ellie's voice cracks, making me realize how much that image of the beach means to her. I finally understand why she always sleeps swaddled in her blue blanket, like a cocoon—warm and happy. Even though I know it's all wrong, I want to give her that moment in the golden sun.

"When you wrote about me in your journal the other day," she says wiping a small tear with the back of her hand wrapped in her black sweatshirt. "When you wrote about me, I knew that I wouldn't die without being known."

My head tilts automatically to the side as my eyes fill with tears, and I bite my lip to keep them from spilling over my lashes.

"When I shared my collage it was like I could finally let people see how I was inside—what I never said out loud before."

All I do is nod my head. On the inside, I tell her that I love her and everything will be OK. There's a part of me that believes it, and there's another part of me that tells me it's all a lie.

"Don't you know better?" Lillie says to me. "You should know better than anyone. You've been diseased for eleven years. You know I'll never let you go. It will never be OK."

*

The kitchen crew must hate us, because they always seem to get something about our orders wrong. They're always missing things from the menu so we have to choose another option, which is a messed-up thing to do to eating-disorder patients. It's wrong on so many different levels. Don't they know how we agonize over having the cinnamon bear crackers or a cookie, or pita bread as opposed to a hamburger bun? Don't they know that it matters, and they can't just change our options at the last minute and expect us not to have anxiety attacks? I plan my meals around certain foods, and if a food isn't available, then my meal has no core and I feel spun off my axis. I don't think the kitchen crew has even met a person with an eating disorder.

The nutritionist and I are not on good terms lately. As I argue and discuss my frustrations with her, she once again says that she has to talk to the head doctor before changes can be made.

"Well, did he die or something? Because it's been almost a week and no one's doing anything."

She leans back with a pout on her face. "He's very busy, but he's reviewing your case."

"In the meantime, though, I'm eating restaurant-size portions of food for every meal."

She's bored with me. "I can assure you that the portions you are eating are normal."

"No, they are not normal," I argue.

"Christen, Americans eat way more than what you're eating. You're on such a low dose of food. You should be thankful, because you should be eating way more."

This freaks me out. There's no way I can eat more. What if she gets pissed and ups my entire food intake just because she can? America is obese. What does she know? She's what my grandma would call "very healthy." I just want her to admit it. I am eating restaurant-size portions. I stand my ground as she walks away. *Just fucking admit it!* I want to scream at her back, but I stand there in silence because I'm afraid she might use her power against me.

After breakfast, I'm allowed to sit in on my evaluation by the staff of the hospital, who discuss my case. The paragraph I wrote explaining my situation is refuted, and I hear things like "You should get more tests on your side pain . . . decreasing food is not the solution . . . she could take a mobility med. . . . what she is eating is normal, 1700 calories a day."

I ascertain that they believe it's my fault my side hurts because of the foods I choose to eat. It just so happens that I'm choosing to eat as much raw food as I can, which means that instead of one hamburger, I have to eat two bowls of salad and almost two cups of vegetables and beans and pita until my stomach feels on the verge of exploding. *Fuck them.* I give up internally and sit silent for the rest of the meeting. When they ask me if that's all I have to say, I nod my head. Here, I have no power.

A little later, in group, we're supposed to meditate to a relaxation tape, but I don't even attempt to listen. Instead, I drift in and out of sleep. They wake me for playgroup, which involves acting out scenes with other people. Ellie and I are partners, and she pretends to be my grandmother offering me fried chicken, potato salad, and cornbread to take home as leftovers. I choose healthfully to take home potato salad and only one piece of cornbread to add to my meal plan. In real life, Ellie would have refused the food or taken it to throw away later. In real life, I would have taken a lot more than necessary and binged on all of it later that night and thrown it up.

I have a hard time dealing with the present-ness of the eating disorder and accepting that for the rest of my life it will be necessary to follow through with the things I presently cannot do. I can answer the questions. I know how I should respond and what I should be doing, what is the right and good thing to do, but I feel like a liar because I can't follow through. In the present, I'm just another patient with an eating disorder I can't control.

Talking to my father on the phone tonight annoys me. I share with him that a huge part of me doubts my ability to function in the real world when I leave this hospital.

He tells me to stop beating myself up. "Isn't overachieving one of your issues?"

One of my issues? This infuriates me. No one's allowed to tell me what my issues are, except those who have degrees in psychology or perhaps other people with eating disorders.

I'm still running the conversation in my head as I rub the toothbrush along my teeth, hard, so it hurts. My eyes look tired and worn. I miss my dreams. I used to look forward to sleep so I could escape myself, but here sleep is short, and restless, and I can't remember dreaming.

It feels like I've closed my eyes for only five minutes when I wake feeling like a truck has run over me. My stomach hurts. I do the shower-and-get-ready thing. I'm bored with carrying my belongings in my arms because I don't have a basket. I'm bored with the plain white tiles and this airless, windowless shower room with its cold floor that hurts my sacrum when I try to do naked sit-ups that are unauthorized anyway. I'm bored with the thud my bare feet make against my towel when I run in place. I'm bored with being here. This disease has reduced me to someone who's compelled to run in place naked in a white-tiled room, so she can try to reduce the anxiety that stems from keeping all this food down and having no one understand.

They say, only when one is sick of the sickness can one be free of the sickness. What does that mean for me? Having been sick and tired and struggling for years, what does that say about me? That I'm not as big a quitter as I thought? That there's something about the sickness I'm not sick of yet? How can this be? I've tried everything.

The voice in the back of my head repeats, "You haven't tried giving up the fear."

In collage group, I'm flipping through magazines, slowly noticing the ways society loves to torture our minds. Sara tells me all the people in the photos are airbrushed to the max. Back when I used to model, I remember the stylists taping clothes to me with duct tape so they fit just so. It's all an illusion, and yet we buy into it as though it's real.

*

Jackie writes on the board:

Restricting anorexia: pride

It makes me feel healthy, thin, worthy, proud.

It's ego-syntonic, meaning we think it's a good thing.

She holds the marker as she writes, her black hair dangling halfway down the back of her blouse. "So, how do you feel when people are trying to make you better and healthy, so you're not anorexic anymore?"

Ellie answers first, in her small distant voice. "Robbed," she says, which sounds in my ears like something worse, like someone was stealing her soul or the air she needed to breathe.

"Misunderstood, rejected, controlled, neglected, caged," we reply.

With her little blue marker Jackie writes all these words on one side of the board, draws a vertical line down the center, and clicks the cap in place. "The dynamic of giving up and eating disorder," she says, "reflects something you struggled with in your childhood." She lets her words sit there for a second before she uncaps her marker again and writes on the other side of the board:

Bulimia: shame

Ego-dystonic

Out-of-control behaviors

To change this disorder brings up something completely different for us. We say words like "worthiness, discipline, and control."

Sara and I look at each other because we understand both sides but gravitate towards the one that makes us feel unworthy all the time and out of control. I glance over at Ellie and suddenly know why it's harder and easier for me to be here. It's harder for me to be here because I feel completely out of control, but it's also easier because I'm bulimic. I have a compelling sense of shame about myself, and I don't want to be this way. But to Ellie, not eating fills her with a sense of pride, and to take that away would be robbing her of something she actually thinks she wants. Both unhappy sides of the same messed-up coin. Pride and shame. And both would destroy us.

*

Sara is still swollen, and they are still doing nothing. "Some people swell ten to fifteen pounds in three days, and depending on the person, it can take months to regulate. But it will regulate," the doctor says.

As I sit in group therapy again I think about the ambiguous phrase "it will regulate." Just the fact that they know so little about eating disorders as a disease makes me apprehensive. It wasn't until the late 1970s that doctors began using the medical terminology *anorexia nervosa.* Eating disorders are like a plague, and the medical establishment deals with them by examining the gravestones instead of digging in and studying the whole body of information that rests underground. We have eating disorders. The doctors should be *studying us* instead of medicating us and telling us that things "will regulate." The system can do better, but I know firsthand that things are not as easy as they seem.

On the couch, Ellie is reading her letter from herself to her eating disorder. "Was I not good enough for you?" she says, and I begin to cry. It reminds me so clearly of that sense of pride I felt when I was thin and in control. As they make me get better, I feel like I failed at being thin, too, and then I feel tricked and angry, because in the end it was all for nothing. The pride and feeling of accomplishment is being taken away. I'm left with the self I loathed—that vulnerable high school girl who couldn't stand up for herself and who wasn't good enough. Except now I'm fat, so I don't have any accomplishment to show for my pathetic little self.

Negative consequences of my ED: (Remember why I want to recover):

1) Poor relationships
2) Fatigue
3) Frustration
4) Depression
5) Guilt/Shame
6) Crazy head (it controls my mind)
7) Anxiety
8) Isolation
9) Can't eat with family
10) Weight gain
11) Low self-esteem
12) Financial difficulties
13) Weight loss
14) Death
15) Chemical imbalance
16) Heart damage
17) Loss of teeth
18) Bad hair

19) Atrophy

20) Cold intolerance

21) Electrolyte imbalance

22) Weakness

23) Isolation from God

24) Loss of concentration

25) Loss of sex drive

26) No motivation

27) Other coping mechanisms

28) Lying/deceit

29) Lacking self-confidence/overly aggressive

30) Keeping secrets (people don't really know me)

31) Fear

32) Rage

33) Education compromised

34) Anger

35) Missing out on activities

36) Causes others pain

37) Self-hatred

38) Low serotonin production

39) Quality of health compromised

40) Insecurity

41) Trouble sleeping

42) Heart palpitations

43) Esophageal tears

44) Amenorrhea

45) Constipation

46) Side pain

47) Worthlessness/lack of accomplishments

48) Chest pain

49) Diarrhea

50) Have to wear kids' clothes

51) Creative thoughts decrease

52) Osteoporosis

53) Feeling fat all the time

54) Suicidal thoughts

55) Distorted body image

56) Unhappiness

57) Irritability/mood swings

As a group, we list fifty-seven negative consequences of our eating disorders. I stare at them on the board in all colors of washable markers wondering why seeing all these horrible things doesn't help me get better. Does it mean I don't fear death? I think it means that a lot of times I'd prefer anything to living in this body and going through fifty-seven negative consequences simply by being the person I can't stop being.

*

Day 27—This is the first time I've counted the days since I was admitted. I was aware of day one and day two, but after that, everything was regulated and controlled, and time disappeared inside one gelatinous bubble. Now it's as if the bubble has burst. Once again, I'm aware of time—just one last day to go until I'm free to leave this place.

At weigh-in this morning, I stand with my back to the digital scale that weighs my progress or failure, depending how I feel about it in the moment. Weigh-ins are never a happy time for us inmates. We're anxious with the horror that they're charting our weight gains, that this is all just a game to make us fatter. The nurses add little marks on a chart they hold at an angle so we can't see. They swoosh us away when we ask any questions, because they know that to reveal even a fraction of weight gain destroys our capacity to function. When I entered the hospital I weighed 116.2 pounds. Today is my last day, so they're allowed to tell me my weight if I want to know.

The nurse looks at the scale and tells me I'm at 119.8 pounds.

In my head I hear the numbers smash into each other—3.6 pounds is my weight gain. "That seems low for the cow-like portions I've been eating. I thought I'd weigh 125 pounds at least."

"That's the point," she says. "To show you that you can eat and be completely satiated without a horrendous weight gain."

I furrow my brow, conflicted about gaining the 3.6 pounds.

The entire time I've been in the hospital I've hated them controlling me, telling me what I must eat, and keeping me from exercising, but now that I'm about to leave and I'll be able to do what I want again, I realize I'm terrified of the freedom. This past month has been the first time since this whole ordeal began that I've kept the food down. This is the first time I've been around people who understand me. This is the first time I've had any hope that I can get better. The outside world holds every opportunity for failure. It's full of people who don't know or understand me. I'm about to be out on my own, and I'll have to count on myself to make sure I'm good. I want to be better, but Lillie is pissed and ready to binge and purge.

I can do this, I tell myself, pushing down the anxiety. *I can stay in control.*

Lillie knows I'm bluffing. She can sense the fear behind my words. "You're pathetic, and you should be afraid, because the only reason you were good was because you were being forced."

That's not true. I'm here of my own free will, which means that I do want to get better.

"Sure," she says, "maybe a part of you does. But we both know what part wins in the end."

Shut up. I don't believe you. I learned stuff here.

She smiles. "We'll see about that. We both know you can't be trusted."

Go away.

"For how long? I do love hide and seek."

When I leave the hospital, I'll take motivation and knowledge with me. I don't need and definitely don't want this disease anymore.

I can be healthy without an eating disorder and move on to better things in my life. Instinctively, now, I hear all the other girls' voices echo in my head, "Yes, you can."

"No, you can't," Lillie laughs. "You always lie."

25

SPIRITUALLY, I STUTTER

My fellow prisoners keep telling me I'm the strong one, but I don't feel strong. I feel broken just like them. However, as I look around the hospital, something within me tastes the sadness here and desperately fights to be free and happy. For the first time, there is a little pinprick opening in my heart. I want something better than oblivion. I'm sick of Lillie's voice in my head making me eat or not eat or run or throw up. She takes away all my happiness and holds me prisoner inside myself. I want to be free.

They say blessed are the cracked, for they let the light in.

At my final group meeting with Jackie, she observes that when I first came here twenty-eight days ago, I was frustrated and scared. She's been watching my progress and says I'll leave the hospital with a sense of happiness and confidence.

"She thinks you're happy and confident," Lillie whispers. "Too bad that's not really you."

Jackie points out how diligently I've worked and contributed to the group. I can see she's right. In spite of my hatred for this place, I've written in my journal every day, spilled my secrets, cried in front of Margaret, kept the food down.

Jackie says something that I believe I will always remember. "No one can ever take away what you accomplished here. No matter what happens in the future, no one can ever take away what you did here."

At first, hearing those words, I feel joy. I've accomplished something. But then her words pierce my heart like the barbs of a dark omen predicting my inevitable failure once I'm outside. Terror.

26

TRACED

Sara and I are sitting at the table next to Ellie, who is working on her treatment plan. She lets out a long breath and holds her papers out to me. "I know I'm not supposed to do this, but what else do you think I should work on?"

My eyes scan the page. "Well, honestly, what I think is important that's not here is something to do with happiness. The question 'what am I going to do now?'"

"What am I going to do now?" Ellie says. "What do you mean?"

"I mean, what are you going to do now? How are you going to deal with what you consider failure, which is you getting better? Because if your eating disorder was happiness for you, then you're going to have to come up with a new definition for happiness."

She opens her binder and shows me what Jackie is making her work on in therapy. "You can read the notebook part there," she says. "It's about the relationship between the eating disorder and myself."

When I take a look at it, the whole list is the negative self-talk that Ellie says goes on all day long in her head. Her two most prominent thoughts: humiliated and disgusted.

"How could people look at me?" she says, as though she's disgusting to look at. Her blue eyes look huge. She tilts her head a little to the left as her blonde bangs cover her eyebrows. "I get angry and depressed when people compliment me."

"Why? What's your first thought when I say you're beautiful?"

"You're such a fucking liar." She looks straight at me.

I'm floored. "Interesting," I say slowly, because I feel the harshness of her reply and the force behind her words doesn't match this tiny blonde pixie that sits next to me on the couch. She tells me how the thoughts go on all day in her head, even if she's having fun. "But sometimes, like today," she says, "it gets so bad I have to go to sleep to make it stop."

The three of us sit around the table as the scissors make a shearing sound. Ellie's cutting through magazine pictures and ripping magazine pages to make me a collage. Sara kneads her blue Silly Putty into small thumb-shaped bowls like pretend pottery.

"How would you like us to respond to that?" I inquire before giving her my feedback.

"I hate pity," Ellie says and rips a magazine page, "and compliments."

"It must have been hard to just sit there and watch someone you love hurt themselves," Sara says.

Ellie and I look at her. We know that we are the people who are being watched, who are hurting ourselves while our loved ones stare on in dismay.

"I'm twenty-five years old," Ellie says, "and I'm just now going to be starting my life, which is depressing and not what I wanted."

"I don't feel like I'm living either," I say.

"But I look at you, and I actually feel depressed because of how much you've accomplished compared to me." She turns to Sara. "And when you talk about how many places in the world you've been."

"It's funny," I interrupt her, "'cause we don't feel accomplished, even though we have all these so-called achievements." Ellie rips another magazine page. My fingers shuffle through the scraps of paper. "I know that all those things are accomplishments according to certain standards, but the real things that make me feel accomplished are things like when Sara remembered that I liked a certain tree on our walk yesterday or when I wrote about you, Ellie, in my journal, and you knew you wouldn't die without being known."

After working on our collages in silence for a while longer we get kicked out of the fish tank and sent back to our room. Ellie takes her evening sleeping pill, and just as I'm about to fall asleep, Sara decides she wants some of the brownies that were on the table in the next room, the psyche room, which is off limits to us because it contains food. She puts on her brown winter coat. Outside the room we hear her say she's going to look for a book. We hear the nurse say she'll help her look. Failed attempt. When she comes back in we offer her our only suggestion, "You can crawl across the hallway," and then burst out laughing. Ellie rolls out of bed groggily and says she'll take a turn. A few minutes later she stumbles back in with a water cup and says the nurse caught her and said, "You know you can't go in there." Ellie had answered, sleepily and drugged, "I want some waaaater." We smile. "So the lady gave me a cup, and here I am." Failed attempt number two.

"What do you think she means?" I ask Sara and Ellie as we sit on our beds. I can't get Jackie's comment out of my head. It had sounded foreboding.

Ellie is telling us about how she spits food. "Even when I'm spitting, I'm still sad," she says, sloppily looking up over her book.

We sit in the silence with that thought for a few moments before Sara, who has been on her bed listening to the conversation, rolls towards us and sighs, "So, what do you think the psyche patients have in their fridge?" We crack up laughing because only those with eating disorders can talk about spitting and throwing up food and want to know what there is to eat. I jump on Sara, and we roll around laughing for a few minutes until the laughter echoes down the hallway and the nurse knocks on our door to tell us we're too loud and we should go to sleep now.

Don't tell me what to do, I think. But I am tired. We turn out our light, and the three of us lie on our beds listening to each other breathe.

"You need to grieve," Ellie says groggily.

"I don't know how," Sara says. "None of us know how, but the answer isn't throwing up in the toilet."

I listen to my breath as I let it out of my chest. "Amen," I add, as though those were the last words in our prayer to God.

We lie in our separate little beds. "I still want a friggin' brownie," Sara says to the darkness, and we all burst out laughing.

27

EXITING THE SAFETY OF PRISON

Today, I am becoming free from the confines of the hospital. With great excitement and even greater fear I'll enter the world and meet my greatest nemesis: myself.

"Hi, my name is Christen," I say for the last time.

"Hi, Christen," I hear back for the last time.

It's nice to have a lot of people use one of their affirmations for me today. Someone says, "I'm going to miss Christen." And we reply, "Yes, you are." And another person says, "I'm going to miss Christen, too." And we reply, "Yes, you are." And my confidence grows. Maybe I will make it. Maybe I'll own the strength that these people see in me. "I love Christen's ass," Sara says. And everyone giggles and replies, "Yes, you do."

Hugging everyone is awkward. The hospital has become my home for the last month, and when I step through the exit doors I'll be out in a world that may not understand me. I'm scared to go.

When they all head to the Overeaters Anonymous meeting, I'm left alone in the hallway. I see Leon walking past the metal gate. He's giddy-giddy with anticipation. I smile. I take in a big breath and make a memory of the hallway, the florescent lights, the long glass fish-tank windows, and the room where for the first time in my life I told people about my eating disorder. I breathe in the little square of grass and the concrete pathway that leads to the metal gate. I step into the hallway and onto the carpet I haven't seen for nearly thirty days. I push against the cool metal of the lobby door that leads to the outside world. Leon takes my little blue suitcase and puts it back in the trunk—déjà vu in reverse.

It's strange being in the real world again. The sun is so bright, and Leon is chatting away. I'm only half listening to what he's saying. "I put Christmas lights up in the boat so it won't be as dark. . . I think Comet's been depressed . . . Cats can pick up on things . . . I'm so happy you're back."

I smile, nod my head, and throw in a comment or two at the right places, but my mind is racing. I feel off balance, now that I've left the safety of the hospital that kept me good—that forced me to be good.

Our car pulls up to the dock. I'm glad to be home. I have the weird feeling I never left. Leon has decorated our boat with white lights around the ceiling of the cabin and colorful lights by our bed, which give the boat a happy glow. As I unpack and put away all my things, Leon and I go through my goals and the contracts I've written. We discuss how he can help me when I have the urge to eat everything and throw it up. The rest of the night I talk about the hospital and Ellie and Sara and tell him some of our inside jokes. Leon laughs. The boat is cold. Leon cuddles me warm. Sleep.

*

My first day of freedom, and I don't like being alone. I make a peanut butter and jelly sandwich thinking, *In your face, dietician.*

Knowing I shouldn't, I look in the mirror. I can see Lillie abhors me. "Disgusting, fat pig," she says in a monotone, and depression sinks in. I observe it, but I don't correct the thoughts, because the pattern of believing her is so engrained.

*

Statistically, most suicide letters are found near or in the bathroom. Most people who kill themselves choose the bathroom to stage the finale. When I learned it was because of the mirrors, it clicked. People want to look at themselves before they die. People want to stare and affirm their self-hatred before they kill themselves off. Mirrors are strange things, magnifying what we focus on, distorting perception. How many hours have I spent in front of one, telling myself I was disgusted with what I saw, telling myself negative and hateful things I'd never say to anyone, even my enemies.

*

Leon and I eat dinner. We talk. At the hospital, one of the things I missed the most was conversation at meals—the ease of other people eating normally and having real conversations, not counting every bite on their forks, not wishing for solitude so they could binge on it all.

Leon and I take turns going through my goals. We discuss how I feel emotionally, physically, and spiritually. We play the affirmation game. My most important affirmation: "I can have a healthy body and not fall back into my eating disorder."

Leon's emphatic answer: "Yes, you can." Here, it makes me slightly uncomfortable, because my marriage hangs on the expectation that I will change.

Sleep brings dreams of buying Skittles for Sara. I wake to the sun shining through the small windows of the v-berth.

As we eat granola, Leon looks at my black '80s-style wristband. Sara, Ellie, two other girls, and I each wear a wristband to symbolize our commitment that this disease will no longer cause us pain.

"You know how I like rituals, right?" I say.

Leon nods.

"Well, one night I led us through a ceremony I made up. We turned off the lights and sat in a circle in the middle of the room. We passed around different objects we'd collected that day on our walk. We drew symbols of protection on each other's forehead with lipstick. We looked in each other's eyes and affirmed the best qualities we saw in one another."

Leon smiles and examines the wristband.

"Sara and I picked these out. They're old-school, but it's all they had at the one store we took a field trip to. I like them. At the end of the ceremony, everyone touched the wristbands as we passed them around the circle, and then we each took one. We put them on and stuck our hands into the middle of the circle, on top of each other like a basketball team or something, and we chanted, 'No more secrets. No more pain. Live free. Live on.'"

"Can I wear it?" Leon asks.

"You can try it on," I say, sliding it off my wrist.

He pulls it over his hand and I cringe a little thinking he might stretch it out and ruin it. He holds his hand up in a fist in front of him.

I laugh, "OK, give it back."

"That's another reason I fell in love with you," he says. "Because you didn't fit in, you're really good at knowing how to make people feel like they're a part of something. I'm sure all the girls still wear their wristbands and think about how cool they are."

I smile and turn the band around my thin wrist.

"You do little things like that all the time. It's always sincere, and that's the kind of stuff that means a lot," he says, "especially for someone with your looks. You could be all snotty, but you're not. Your personality doesn't match your looks."

This is funny, as in puzzling, because I don't think I'm pretty. I think I'm average.

"You're hot," Leon says, and half winks at me.

Ha. That's the most amusing part. Who in their right mind would ever in a million years categorize me as hot?

28

MY HARD LIFE

The night creeps over, after the purple sunset, and melts the sky into lavender watercolor clouds. On the same bench where two old men feed the birds each morning, I sit alone with the glow from my iPod shinning through my pants pocket, like I'm smuggling a flashlight. A little bit ago I looked in the mirror and saw my fat ass and got pissed.

Leon asked, "Why are you always so moody?"

I put on my headphones and decided to leave before I said something I'd regret.

"I'm going to go get a latte at the coffee shop."

"Are you going to stay there for a while?"

"Yeah, probably. I'm going to go write in peace where you won't make me feel like a bitch."

He says something like "Yeah, go write" and "You are a bitch" and the comment that I remember verbatim, "You act like you have a hard life."

*

I know I'm slipping. I thought Leon and I were going to have a nice, happy dinner at the Kettle. My stomach has felt like an overstuffed jelly doughnut all day long. At dinner, all I want to eat is a honey bran muffin and a cup of onion soup.

"You're restricting," Leon says and gives me that annoyed face.

"I'm saving room for the Ben & Jerry's ice cream I have at home," I say.

"Stop trying to justify and rationalize it because you have Phish Food at home."

I'm not trying to justify anything. I'm just full. I'm trying not to overdo it, because I want to be comfortable and enjoy my night rather than spending it focusing on not throwing up.

He says, "I'm sick of how our sex life suffers and how you have no confidence in your body. Right now I wish you were just normal or that I could fix you or something."

"I ordered exactly what I wanted for dinner because I know my side pain issue. I know my own body, despite what others think."

We sit in silence.

I say, "So, what now? You're not going to talk to me?"

"I have nothing to say." He takes a bite of his burger.

I mutter, "Eff you," and scan the room.

*

Our footsteps along the pavement are all I hear on our way back to the car. I don't talk at all on the drive home because I'm trying to convince myself of all the reasons I don't want to throw up. I ordered a second muffin just to appease him, but the extra food presses into my stomach until it feels like a balloon that's about to pop.

In the moment of feeling too full, if my anxiety is triggered, then it's easy to refute logical arguments against purging.

Oh, I may rupture my esophagus.

Nah, that won't happen. Look at how many times I've done it before.

I should sit down and breathe, draw a picture, listen to music, take a walk, write down all fifty-seven horrible things this eating disorder has done for me.

Boring.

I should tell myself that Lillie can't control me, that just this one purge is not the way towards having a happy life. Besides, it's never just once.

But just do it this once.

It's like giving an addict just a little heroin, just a small drink, just a little bit too much food in the stomach. The threat of sudden death never scares me when I'm triggered. There is nothing anyone can say to calm me down. I'm a smart, rational, and logical person but Lillie is now in control. All day long she thinks about food, about being thin.

In the past, I planned my binges like I'd plan vacations. When I'm triggered, the planning starts.

She begins to talk to me. Us. "First, let's go to the grocery and get ice cream, bread, peanut butter cups, and Alfredo sauce and then to the donut shop and get bear claws, sugar puffs, iced chocolate donuts, and custard-filled ones and say they're for coworkers. Pick them out slowly and carefully, so we look held together and peaceful. Then, let's hit up Taco Bell and Jack-in-the-Box and go home and turn on the TV and eat till we're full and throw up, come back, eat, and throw up again."

I shake my head to try to disengage Lillie's voice.

Leon watches my internal struggle, and I see his disappointment. I watch him watch the road, purposely not looking at me.

I can't stop thinking about the pressure in my stomach as I keep trying to convince myself I'm fine.

He asks, "How are you feeling?" and I say, "Annoyed. I'm overfull," and we sit in silent hatred.

Before I go to sleep, I call Julie. I'm silently focusing on my hatred when she suddenly shares, "Leon was at my house when you were in the hospital. He was telling me that when he married you, he knew you were the only one for him. And then, being completely away from you, he felt it just as strong. He said he'd do anything to make you better." The words hit me hard, as though she's whipped her cell phone at the side of my face. "He's cute. You're lucky to have him," she says.

"Eat a little ice cream," Lillie says.

Get rid of it. Bad. Bad. Bad.

In the morning my throat hurts a little. I feel guilty. Drink water. Brush my teeth.

*

Friday night, when I come home from work, Leon is depressed. He says he pretends all the time to be OK, but sometimes he thinks about all the negative.

"What negative," I ask.

"It's about everything," he says.

But the truth is that it's about me and how I'm not passionate. Maybe I could try drinking alcohol. Drunk people seem to want sex. But I know better than to force myself to diversify. "Diversifying addictions just gives us more ways to kill ourselves," Sara once said. "It's an insult to our intelligence."

Leon said:

He's unhappy.

He's been sweeping it under the rug for a year and a half.

Our marriage lacks passion.

He really wants a kid.

Even if I did have a kid, I'd be an unfit mother.

The disease has taken so much from him.

If I feel fat now, then what would my mental state be like if I were pregnant?

He's been wondering if I'm in love with him. He thinks I love him but I settled, because if I were in love with him nothing else would matter.

He can't touch me, because I feel gross when I'm touched.

I love food more than him.

I'm selfish.

*

Of course, the logical thing to do is not what I do. What happens instead?

When Leon goes to sleep, I go to the kitchen and eat crackers, peanut butter, and ice cream. I throw it up into a large bowl. Painstakingly, so as not to make noise, I dump it overboard, then panic when I realize it's sitting there, floating. I scoop it into the empty ice cream container and dump it into the public trashcan at the docks, the whole time watching for movement on the boat. When I close the door again, safely back inside, I rinse the bowl. I hear movement. I freeze like a rabbit with a gun pointed directly at its heart. Then

I hurt my neck jumping over to the couch, so I can pretend to be peacefully watching TV and drinking blue Gatorade.

When he opens the door, his look says he knows, but he feels the need to torture me with words. "Don't try to hide it, I smell the vomit," he says, "and I see the bowl you're trying to hide."

I hold my breath, fixate on the TV, and grip the plastic Gatorade bottle till my hand is white and he shuts the door and leaves me alone.

I hate him. He is my trigger.

I sleep on the couch and cry about us and think about divorce and go through the pros and cons in my head. *It's not fair to him to stay with me. If we did get a divorce, who would want me? My life now would be over.* I cry about how he says he has a retirement plan for us. I cry about Sara, who says she wants to kill herself when she feels there will be no end to this. I want to slice myself with a knife, can't, want to drink, won't, don't want to throw up anymore, but stopping is not what I choose, even though my throat hurts and I don't enjoy it. I cry myself to sleep with Lillie's arms wrapped around me.

I go into the v-berth only as Leon leaves for work. No words are exchanged.

*

My mom is on the list of people who don't understand. When I get off the phone with her, I'm crying. I've made her cry, because I told her that I don't want to talk anymore. She sniffled, "OK, just know I love you."

Why do conversations end like this? What triggers my desire to disconnect? She called and asked how my marriage is doing and how sex has been since I came home from the hospital. "That's an important part of a marriage," she said, "and if you don't give him that, then…. Love…" *Blah, blah, blah.* "Do you want him to leave?"

My mind contemplates and pulls both ways.

"Did the hospital focus on that at all?"

"No," I said, "it dealt with the more important fact that I throw up food."

I don't want to talk to her, because she doesn't get it. She loves me and has only good intentions, but she tells me the stories I write are a tad depressing and asks me why I'm high and low and wants to know if I should be on medication.

Intimacy.

Love.

Me. Leon. Lillie.

What am I always doing wrong?

Lillie whispers, "You know what he did wrong. He married you."

*

Leon and I are talking about the half-empty, half-full glass analogy. In the argument, I somehow have become the glass.

Leon says, "It's like I have a glass, but the things I want won't fit."

He's talking about the things he wants from the marriage that I can't provide because I'm a mess.

I say, "So why don't you go find another glass?"

"Because I want this one."

"Well, then, accept that you can't fit things in." *I suck. Leon loves me. I love Leon. I hate myself. We both agree we hate Lillie. If I could kill her without harming myself, I would.*

He's not irrational for wanting me to be normal.

*

Note to self—

I am not crazy. I am not a freak. I am not a failure. I am not a bad person. I am getting better. I am not alone. There are correlations between the eating disorder and sex. I am not the only one. I am good enough as is. I will deal with the eating disorder first. I am the most important person. I am not alone. I am not a freak. I am not a freak. Will anyone besides the hospital girls ever understand me? Even if no one does I am still not a freak, and I am not alone. Do you hear that, self? Say it again. Say it again. Say it again and again and again. Until you believe it.

The pattern is the same. The energy between us has become more unhappy and hostile. Leon has become increasingly depressed as a result. I feel like a rat trapped in a bell jar being watched from all angles, having my space constantly invaded.

I often wish I could substitute alcohol as my numbing method, but even when a little wine makes me numb out to the sex I give him, I realize my addiction, my personal poison, lies in what I can stuff into my stomach and regurgitate on cue.

Today, I didn't make a meal plan, because I hate them. I just want to be able to eat what my body wants to eat. When I go to make more salad, Leon gives me the disapproving look that shows his lack of faith in me. It's written all over his silent face.

The sleeves of my shirt hide dry soybeans from him, until he makes me show him where I'm getting them. He pulls at my sleeves, gives me the glare, and walks away.

I just wanted a handful of soybeans. I know they're not on my meal plan. I feel guilty for eating them, because I'm conditioned to hear something that will trigger me... When he says, "You're still hungry," what I hear him saying is, "Now, I think you are throwing up."

He leaves to smoke a cigar.

I get in my car and drive away from the boat with the intention of binging. It's the first time since I left the hospital that I'm purposely going to buy food to throw up.

"Failure. A Failure. You are a failure," Lillie chants it singsong.

When the anger comes, I do it anyway. For the cream puffs and doughnuts, I pay cash. I put tampons and water on the credit card. Then I sit in the dark street, in the car, eating. But instead of the high, there is emptiness and a rush of pure rage when it doesn't taste good and it doesn't make me feel better like it used to.

Where do I go when my numbing method doesn't numb?

As I'm throwing up in the restroom of the nearest fast food place, Leon calls twice.

On the third call, I pick up. "I don't want to talk," I say, and hang up.

As the toilet flushes, I feel like a pathetic failure, enraged and disgusted at myself for not having the discipline to work out and restrict.

Choose one: eating disorder or sex.

You choose.

I contemplate taking a bottle of laxatives but it's not my style. Hating myself, on the other hand, has become my style. I do it well. Hate myself for failing like this, for buying food, wasting money. *Fucking self. Fucking weak, pussy self. Fuck you, you fucking bitch.*

Finally I drive home and tiptoe my way to bed. I fall asleep with an old friend running her hands along my hair. *Hate life. Want to die.*

29

THE CIRCLE I DIDN'T CLOSE

The days are mostly bad with a few good days in between. On the good days, I feel proud of myself, in control, and somewhat at peace. On the bad days, I wish I wasn't married. Last night was a good night. I was so happy to be with Leon. I don't understand why the happiness didn't carry into today.

I ask him what's wrong, and he says he's just tired. That's a lie. I call him on it, so he says, "I feel unappreciated for last night and today and for my hard work."

Last night, when I came home from work, he had wine and strawberries ready, and we ate soup and salad and salmon that he'd prepared, and he gave me a massage. We showered together, took a walk, got dessert, and watched a movie. This morning, he cleaned the boat and did our laundry.

My guilt and the anger compete with each other. *What do I have to do to show you I appreciate it?* What should I have done? Am I preoccupied with my own thoughts again, being selfish, not thinking of others? What am I doing wrong?

I am better than this. I am so much better than this.

The sad thing is that last night I was so happy with all his efforts—his massage and our walk and spending time together. My heart was full.

Tonight, like a bipolar wife, I once again find myself wishing I weren't married to him, so I could have my own life and no one to please.

Acne is supposedly an external sign of repressed anger. I've been breaking out since last week. Is that a coincidence? I've started to get depressed again. Depression is rage turned inwards. Less water, more coffee, more Lillie, more stress, more sense of failure, more feeling fucked up. Sometimes I hate everything.

I feel fat and ugly. I'm not pretty anymore. My clear skin was the main thing I liked about myself, but now that's gone. I also like my eyebrows, because they're full, and my clavicle, because it juts out and makes me look svelte. But people notice skin. They notice if you're scarred, if you're flawed. They notice when you don't look young anymore. Maybe, finally, my skin decided to expose how I've felt for years on the inside—ugly and flawed. Maybe, I just decided it was time to turn inside out, bring the ugly to the outside, so the inside finally can be at peace.

*

Leon wakes me to go to church. I don't go. I'd rather sleep. Church has only made me feel guilty for my failures. I'm angry. I now sort of believe in reincarnation. It's the best way I can come to terms with my life. Somehow I must be here to work out something.

When Leon gets back from church we can't decide what we'd like to do, so we wash clothes. Flipping through the hamper to consider my choices— sweatpants and t-shirts, which I pretty much live in, along with a sweatshirt because I'm perpetually cold—he says that I always look like a bum.

"It would be nice, not if you dressed up, but if you looked decent at least," he says. He's noticed the only time I dress up is when I'm going out with Sara.

Hello? I'm cold all the time. We live on the ocean. Plus, I hate dressing up. Why is it such a big deal?

His comments make me feel like shit. I can't just be myself. I feel pressured to dress up and be someone I don't feel like being to please him. If he wanted to dress like a bum all the time, I'm pretty sure I'd let him. As long as he was happy, what the hell would I care what he looked like? He met me when I lived with my parents in Hawai'i, where it's always eighty degrees, and my staple wardrobe consisted of skirts and tank tops over my bathing suit.

I'm feeling frustrated, defeated, and unloved, as though the real me doesn't matter as long as I look good on the outside. Society is so obsessed with image.

Stupidly, I bought in to the obsession.

"But I'm not happy," I say.

Lillie answers, "But you're skinny," and somehow that justifies the torture. My worth as a human being has been reduced to one criterion—skinny.

At Leon's insistence I'm still going to therapy sessions. I'm angry about it, about the part where I have to pay a hundred dollars an hour to hear myself explain my own life.

Despite the apology letter he gave me this morning, I've checked out. All day I binge like a machine that's programmed to go through the motions. I eat and throw up bacon biscuits, two bagels and chai, coffee, doughnuts. I spit two burgers. I throw up chocolate, noodle soup, and frozen pizza . . . I feel drained, empty, and lifeless—one breath away from tipping over onto the sidewalk and not getting up. I've wasted my whole day and binged away the money I earned at work. I'm enraged at myself. I want to starve . . . sleep for a few days . . . it hurts . . . my eyelids are heavy . . . my neck hurts. I'm nauseated. Nothing makes me happy now.

Lillie fails me, and Leon doesn't want me. He has to struggle to have patience with me every day. That sucks, the fact that my husband has to endure being with me every night.

I feel sick. I need . . . What the hell do I need? . . . Gatorade? . . . A lobotomy? . . . Peace? . . . To cry out all this pain and shame and frustration? . . . My glands are swollen. Why am I such a weak, stupid addict? *I hate you, Christen. I hate you . . . No, I'm even too tired to hate you. I'm just so disappointed* . . . I want to go back to when I was a little kid, when I felt happy and good enough, when the days were fun. Now my life is a morbid game of impossible expectations.

I try so hard, yet I fail so aggressively. It's impossible for a normal person to understand the compulsion to drive to a fast-food restaurant and binge and throw up in the bag.

I thank God after I remember that I left the bag in the kitchen sink and I still have time to throw the evidence away before my husband comes home and finds it. It's sick. It's horribly, massively sick, and I don't even know why I do it anymore. I'm terrified by my inability to stop. I'm tired of being a warrior who's always losing. I'm exhausted with being a failure.

30

THE LOWEST BIRTHDAY

It was selfish for me to get married and drag Leon down to my level of hell. I loved him more than any other man I'd ever met, but did I somehow think that his love would save me from myself?

When I was a little kid, my mom used to read me my favorite bedtime story. It was about a little duck egg that was all alone on the top of a mountain. One day, when the egg hatched, a little duckling peeked out at the great big world and realized he was all alone. My mom thought it was cute when my eyes got big and sad and I was almost scared. I'd ask, "He's all alone?" as if somehow it couldn't be true. Most of my life I felt like that little duckling looking around at the great big world and thinking I was all alone. It began to feel normal.

Sometimes I wonder if that's why it's so hard to kill Lillie. Maybe without her I'd have to admit that I'm scared of being alone.

Happy Thanksgiving, Lillie. My birthday falls on Thanksgiving week, which means there will be too much food. I'll lack self-control, no matter how hard I attempt to be good and stable.

The weekend festivities go as predicted. I'm able to be good for a short time, until inevitably I eat a few bites too much and lose control. The day after Thanksgiving, when I go back to work, the cycle continues. It's easier to continue hurting myself when I already feel like a worthless failure.

Leon calls me when my shift is supposed to end and asks me when I'm coming home. "On my way," I lie, as I get in my car and head to the drive-thru. On the short ride home I inhale the milkshake. I sip the last drop as I pull into my parking stall at the dock.

Leon is walking up the ramp. He smiles and waves when he sees me.

I muster a smile back while dropping the empty cup on the floor. I hurry out of the driver's seat and meet him on the sidewalk. He's carrying his towel and shower bag, and I turn with him and walk to the bathhouse, trying to remain friendly but aware of the mounting urge to throw up the milkshake as soon as possible. When he realizes that I have been walking with him not to keep him company but because I want to go to the bathroom, the sadness on his face crushes my heart. He knows me well enough to know what I'm doing. I hate him sometimes, because only he is aware of all my tricks.

After I throw up, instead of trying to correct my behavior and start over, my sick mind takes a different path. *OK, he's in the shower, which means I have a few minutes to eat something else.* As my mind races, I slide open the wooden door of the boat, and step over the platform, down the stairs, into the belly of our house. And my heart *stops*. The boat is full of purple streamers and white balloons.

The air feels heavy in my lungs, as I reach tentatively towards the ceiling as though the balloons will explode at my touch. I turn each one delicately as the words written in Leon's handwriting fall into my heart:

I will love you forever.
A picture of a *shaka* sign (a Hawaiian greeting symbol)
Leon and Christen 4'Eva.
I love you more than sour gummie worms.
You are beautiful.
I love your ass (and a picture of a girl with an ass).
You complete me.
A picture of a sunflower.
Happy Birthday
You are a sunflower (my symbol of strength).
I love to hear you smile.

You deserve the best.
Jesus has plans for you.
Jesus loves you.
You will be a famous writer.
I'm always here for you.
You are my best friend.
You are my dream girl.

Tremendous guilt slumps me down against the couch and sobs overtake me. *God, please help me. I'm such a horrible person.* The balloons hover around me with their promise of the wonderful life I don't deserve. How does anyone love an addict who lies and breaks promises?

Leon loves me so much. Now I understand why his face was so sad when he went to take a shower. He was calling me to tell me to come home because, while I was buying the milkshake, he was decorating the boat and writing love notes to me on little white balloons with purple streamers. While I was throwing up, he knew what was waiting for me in the boat. My heart collapses.

When the boat rocks, I know Leon has stepped on deck, and I frantically wipe my eyes. When he walks in I'm holding a balloon and trying to form words without crying.

"What's wrong?" he asks.

"It's so pretty. Thank you." That's all I can muster without completely going to pieces. "I love it," I say, when what I mean is, "I wish I deserved this."

31

EVERY PARTICLE ASPIRES TOWARDS ITS BOUNDARY

As Christmas passes, I want to understand myself, be at peace, and not have my disease. Both weekend days are bad days for the eating disorder. The familiar hopelessness creeps in, and I hear Jackie telling me as I left the hospital, "No matter what happens, no one can take away what you did here." I hear another girl's voice, too, as she told me, "You are the strong one." But I feel weak.

I don't want to let anyone see the raw part of myself, so I camouflage it like a tiger trap. There's no warning, no halfway in. Once I take a step, I fall and see just how deep the hole goes.

32

HOME AGAIN, HOME AGAIN, JIGITTY JIG

By a twist of events and mishaps Leon and I make our way back to Hawai'i. I'm suddenly elated that I get to return to where I believe all my happy memories reside.

When we finally touch down, the airport smells like plumeria flowers, and my mom and dad are all smiles as they greet us.

Leon had scoped out our new apartment complex on Craigslist before we left California, and my parents had picked an apartment for us, so we'd have a place to move into as soon as we came back.

I had asked my parents not to put anything in it. I was so excited to decorate my first actual home. I had lain awake at night in California trying to picture what our apartment was going to look like and how I would decorate it. I'd thought maybe I'd make tie-dye curtains out of white sheets and door separators out of shells and yarn.

When my parents take us to our new apartment, I see they've decorated with curtains and blinds and bathroom stuff, as well as a couch and other furnishings they found. They're excited and smiling, but my heart drops, and I have to hold back tears. They know a friend is coming to visit us in less than a week, so they don't want us to be stressed about getting silverware and curtains, but the sight of my new house decorated in my absence makes me feel torn between gratitude and selfishness.

I smile on the outside while fury rages internally. I had asked them only one thing: "Please do not put anything in my house." *They couldn't even respect my one wish? Does my opinion not stand for crap? Why am I not taken seriously? I stood up for myself, said what I wanted, even threatened 'You'd better not,' and in the end it didn't matter. I have no power even when I use my voice.*

They say if I hate it I can take everything down and they won't care, but I don't think that's true. I almost burst into tears as I look at their happy, expectant faces. Leon and I agree to go to church with my parents the next evening, and they go home.

Most of my life, I've given in to someone else by playing the good little girl and letting my wishes be trampled. As I walk around the apartment, I realize my war for independence was fought with the only thing I could control, my body.

*

As I sit in church, I begin to think the air conditioner is trying to freeze me alive. By the time the service ends, I have a migraine. I feel like I'm going to hurl as we begin the short walk back to my parents' house.

While I'm in the kitchen eating a bagel, I begin to open the lid of a plastic container of chili, and my dad calls out, "Eating again?" with that disapproving tone, like I'm being watched and monitored.

"All I had was a bagel," I say.

"You have to want to help yourself," he says.

Eff you. I throw the lid back on the container and leave it on the counter, grab my things, and walk out the door, telling Leon as I pass by, "I want to go home now."

"Bye," my dad says.

I want to say, *Fuck you. I wasn't thinking about throwing up. I felt like crap, and all I wanted to do was eat something to stop my head from pounding.* Instead, I let my parents' door bang loudly, walk up the stairs to the driveway, and lie on the cement next to our car until Leon comes and unlocks the door.

"Come on," he barks.

I slither into the passenger seat and stare out the window as we ride home in silence. Without a word, I brush my teeth and go straight to bed. He doesn't say goodnight to me and makes no effort to be quiet while changing the light bulbs in the kitchen. He doesn't like us going to bed angry.

*

Lately, I notice that being home again brings my family to the tip of my fingers, which is both nice and confrontational. My mom and I have been hanging out—taking walks to the pool, to the health food store, to get shave ice. As a family we go to the beach and have family dinners that usually involve lots of laughter. Hawaiʻi is my happy place, where I feel more alive, where I'm out in open air, and where I'm motivated and content.

The unexpected confrontations chip away at my heart. Pieces peel away like tiny paint flecks. The cracks occur at simple moments, like when I watch my mom excitedly prepare food and see how happy she is to spend time with us as a family. At her dinners, I force myself to keep the food down, because it hollows me out to throw up her love. I've kept food down out of respect for others and the connection to the labor and the love that went into it. However, it's always easy to throw up junk food that I buy at a big supermarket with no face attached to it.

Life is full of monotonous workdays that go exactly the same. All day I anticipate the great plans I've made for after I get off work, but by the time I finish, the life has been sucked out of me, and I just want to eat dinner and watch TV like a mindless zombie.

Lillie has figured out I've been evading her, but she always wins at hide-and-seek. Leon confronts it. "I know you've been struggling lately. I think you'll always struggle with it unless you make up your mind not to."

There's nothing to say that won't get us into an argument, so I stay silent and let the hatred seethe. I hate that he knows the darkest parts of me.

Since I hurt my knees in Germany, I can't run like I used to. My knees can handle only about twenty minutes of the impact before I have to stop, angry and frustrated. How can I be skinny if I can't burn calories?

Someone tells me about yoga. "It would be good for your knees."

"Yeah, thanks. I'll look into it." I'm too ashamed to ask how many calories I could burn by taking a class. Even though I hated it, I miss being able to run. *Fine. I'll try yoga.*

Bikram yoga brings out my competitive nature. For starters, I'm looking at a full-length mirror for a full ninety minutes. I find myself feeling slightly elated when someone has to lie down in corpse pose because she needs a rest. It's mean, I know, but it makes me feel stronger. Even though the teachers say we're supposed to focus only on ourselves, it's impossible not to see everyone else in my peripheral view and either feel proud during a pose, because I'm prettier, or embarrassed because I'm not as graceful, flexible, or thin as someone else.

I try to focus only on myself, but I always compare myself to the best girl in the room. On the days that I can appreciate my body, I feel like I win. On the other days, when I find myself saying nasty things to myself, I fail. As I breathe deeply through my nose, I can't help but think of Snow White and the evil queen. *Mirror, mirror on the wall, who is the fairest of us all?*

*

Leon and I sit down to watch a movie after dinner. I eat my large cookie and then take my pint of ice cream out of the freezer.

"The cookie wasn't enough?"

"Eff you," I almost whisper.

He moves into a long-ass monologue, "It bothers me constantly, how you're not honest. I never see you even attempting progress."

"What the hell? You can't even begin to know what it's like to be in my head. How dare you say that? My life right now is leaps and bounds of progress from the constant anxiety of just wanting to eat and puke, eat and puke *all* day long."

He's still talking, but I've stopped listening. His mouth keeps moving, but all I hear is *blah, blah, blah.*

Leon's acting out the same mechanisms my father uses: not validating my feelings, trying to control everything and its outcome, directing everything his way, pretending he understands when he doesn't. The difference between the two is that Leon leaves me a message the next day explaining how he's analyzed the situation and made a list of how he could have responded better during our argument. This is different than the way my dad and I interact by ignoring each other, as though one person's silence will smoke the other person out. Instead, Leon always comes back to me having analyzed his behavior for his own understanding and the betterment of our relationship.

33

SPIN DOCTOR

After a mellow workday, my dad and I meet at my parents' house, and I hand over my car keys so he can drive to Chili's. We get a booth with an overhanging tin light that streams yellow and reminds me of a bug zapper on the marshlands. We talk about Zack and his grizzly man beard, which my dad calls slovenly but I like. Over nacho cheese I load jalapeños onto my chip and tell him that both Zack and I now believe in reincarnation.

"Get this," he says. "I told Zack he was a spin doctor, and he said, 'Who do you think I get it from?'" My dad gets excited and passionate as he says, "You see what he did? He spun what I said!" Then he vents some frustrations about my mom, and I find it ironic that each thinks it's the other one that's difficult.

"Why do you think you're dark?" he asks, and then adds, "You're not."

I sigh, take a breath, and begin, "This is what you do. Don't tell me how I feel. Just validate that I feel depressed. Just let me be depressed."

"That's wrong thinking, and you are what you think, so you have to change your thinking." After a bit more argument, he finally says, "Fine. Be depressed."

For the first time I get it—why he doesn't validate me. He is and always has been the guru. His concept of the power of the mind has never allowed Zack and me to have the wrong thoughts about anything. He was trying to teach us to free ourselves from the mind's power, because he saw our infinite potential.

Ha. He wouldn't validate me, because he wouldn't allow me to be anything less than what he saw.

*

Yesterday was a bad day with the eating disorder. The cravings consumed me, and the only thing that could calm my mind was my mouth's constant motion. Last night, I opened and closed the fridge door a bazillion times, thinking each time that something new and delicious would appear, something that would satisfy me completely. Top-shelf happiness, right next to the eggs. Who knew? But nothing satisfied me, so finally I opted for sleep.

The next day, I'm dehydrated, and the yoga room hits me like a hot brick. The teacher is pushing to hold the postures longer, and I have to lie down. When I try to get up, dizziness and nausea overtake me. I frantically fumble out of the hot room and flop on the bench outside. Everything is woozy and going dim as stars and dots come into focus. I clench the bench and panic. *Don't pass out. Please, please, don't pass out here all alone. Oh, God, I need to throw up.* One of the instructors finds me on the bathroom floor hugging the toilet seat gagging up air. "Drink a coconut water," she says. "Don't worry the heat gets to everyone at some point." But I know the truth about why I'm hugging the toilet. *Why did I think I could get away with binging yesterday? I was even planning to binge again today. Stupid.*

For the rest of the day, I cycle through bouts of wooziness and nausea and a dull but constant headache. The scare in the yoga studio causes me to pack a big lunch, eat it all, and keep everything down.

One of the reasons I practice Bikram yoga is that it forces me to keep all my electrolytes in my body. It scares me into treating myself like a normal person. The pathetic reality settles in. I desperately need something to scare the shit out of me on a daily basis in order to stay on track.

*

After work, I massage my temples to get rid of my headache and walk around the corner to the therapist's office. This is my third time seeing her, but I still haven't made up my mind if I like her. She's passive. She has me lie on the couch and then takes me through a relaxation and into a scenario where I visualize a cave. In the middle of the cave is a desk, and on the desk she says there is something waiting for me.

"What is it?" she asks.

"I can't see it," I say, squinting. "There's an old jewelry box on the desk. It's white with blue inside. It has a little plastic ballerina like the one I had in my jewelry box when I was a kid. When I'd open the box, she would twirl on her toes in front of her little mirror."

"Open the jewelry box," she says.

In the cave, I bend down and catch sight of my eye reflected in the small mirror. Something about my eye is so sad. On the couch, tears drop sideways down my cheeks, and my throat curls up in a tight flower bud.

She continues unperturbed, "There's a paper in the box with a message for you. Take it out and read it."

My hands remove the small paper scroll and unroll it. "You are enough," I read out loud. As I say those words, tears stream down my face. I feel as though God is saying them directly to me.

"OK, it's time to say goodbye," she says. "This place will always be here when you want to visit."

As I close the wooden door to the cave, I watch prisms of light leap through the forest, and then I'm back on her couch. She smiles peacefully, but when I leave her office I'm filled with more questions than answers.

Two days pass. I dissect the experience until, finally, I have my weekly meeting with my other therapist who specializes in cognitive behavioral therapy.

"Please, just tell me what it means," I say.

My cognitive therapist and I dance around terms and feelings and eventually she explains some possible answers. The light sparkling through the trees represents the truth that I can't fully grasp yet. Behind the door lie the answers I seek, but I'm afraid of finding them because then I'll have to change.

"It's okay," she says, seeing me slump back on the couch. "We all hold on to what's familiar. It's like being in a river holding onto a log to stay afloat. If you're going to swim towards the unknown shore, you have to completely let go of the log you know so well."

I nod with a frown.

"Let's move on to your homework."

I open my notebook. "What do I restrict in my life? What does it offer me? What does it take away? Overall, I realized that I restrict two main things in my life: food and sex. When I wrote out what they offered, the answers were the same: power, safety, control, and detachment. I never realized before that I thought about those two things in the same way. What do you think that means?"

"What do you think it means?"

I don't answer because what I hear in my head is, *You are sicker than you thought.*

She begins to repeat back to me all the strengths I see in the fifteen-year-old girl I used to be, but I'm zoning out. I feel like crying. I remember the time in the hospital when I told Ellie she was beautiful.

"You're such a fucking liar," she said.

My eyes glaze over blankly as I focus on the clock ticking on the wall behind my therapist. When I had that conversation with Ellie, I couldn't understand why she wouldn't see the good in herself. Now I know why she responded so harshly. She couldn't allow herself to think she was good, because it hurt too much to be disappointed, because as much as she wanted to believe she was pretty, the inner voice always told her she was ugly.

*

In the elevator on the way back to my car, I hold my validation ticket with the two green stickers. My therapist keeps the stickers in her top drawer. I stare at my morphed reflection in the closed doors. "You're such a fucking liar," I say letting it linger. The bell dings, and I smile politely as a well-dressed woman enters. I wonder if she can feel the vibration of my words. *Mirror, mirror on the wall, who's the fairest of them all?*

34

MAINTAINING EQUILIBRIUM

When night finally comes, I tell Leon I'm going to the store to get ice cream, and I'm not going to be good. Why lie about it anymore? I'm so exhausted with playing this game of pretending to be someone I'm not. I'm an addict, and I need the ice cream. I need to eat it and throw it up, so that I can be done and over this craving.

In the hospital, Jackie had walked us through an exercise involving a trip to the grocery store to buy binge food. We'd revealed the twenty different decisions we make when we decide to go to the store. She'd told us, "At every step of the way you can make a different decision to stop the process of the binge no matter what step you are at." She had paused for dramatic effect. "You could stay home, you could not buy the ice cream, and you could not eat the ice cream once you have it at home."

Like that's going to happen.

When I'm actually in a binge state, good decisions are like white noise. I can't think or see anything but what I want, and I will blow through all the roadblocks to get it. I can tell myself, *OK, self, you don't have to go to the store.* Lillie yells, "Shut up! Get out of my way or I'll run you over." Sometimes Lillie whispers, "Come on, you know you want it. I'll take care of it for us. Don't worry about it." And pretty soon I'm home with a large spoon diving into a gallon tub of ice cream.

If I had kept this binge a secret, it would have continued for days instead of just one night.

Leon doesn't get it. He ignores me for the next two days, saying that I've taken this to a whole new level by doing it in front of him.

You don't even know how many levels I can take this.

We ignore each other. The house is silent.

My stomach has been in pain for the past two weeks. Every obligation makes me anxious. Everything stresses me out like a clock constantly ticking in the background.

Perhaps I'm better off alone, as Lillie leads me to believe, with no one to drag down. Whatever I choose to do affects no one else but me.

Leon finally talks to me. He brings up the ice cream binge the other night. He tells me that I contributed nothing to the conversation and didn't validate his feelings at all. It's all true. I am the master of numbing myself to get out of a conversation when I don't want to be there.

To Leon, I shrug as I pull off my sweaty yoga t-shirt.

He nearly cries, which breaks through my armor. "If something happens to you one day, I don't want to look back and know that I just sat here on the couch and watched you."

I have no answer.

"I love you, and I still want to be with you," he says. "Do you still want to be with me?"

Maybe I'll learn the hard way. Maybe I'll die. "Sometimes I just want to be alone," I say. I think he'd be happier without me. Sometimes I want to say, "No, I don't want you to be here. I want to be alone," but deep down I know I'd regret losing him.

"If you don't want to be with me, just let me know. It will hurt, but I will walk out that door," he says.

I leave the house. As I drive away, I listen to Ani DiFranco. And I cry and cry, hard and heavily into the space between me and the steering wheel. *All the guilt. All the time. All the money. All the relationships I've wasted. While people starve, I manipulate. I have secrets, I'm dirty and shameful. I lie. I'm a bad person.*

What does it offer me? What does it offer me? I think it over and over until the answer comes like a bug splattering against my windshield. It allows me to gag the voice that says, "You are nothing, you are nothing, you are nothing." It allows me to forget that I hate myself.

*

Worthless. That seems to be the word of the day today in therapy. As we talk, the larger underlying theme we circle is my subconscious belief that I'm worthless. It's the root of everything, including why I like helping people . . . It's validating . . . Why I feel better when I'm alone . . . I don't have to give my energy to anyone . . . Why I brush aside conversation about me and direct the conversation back to the other person . . . I don't feel I'm important . . . Why I downplay my good qualities . . . Deep down, I feel I'm worthless, and my self-confidence is severely lacking.

*

I'm unhappy. Big surprise.

Leon looks at the salad I've made and asks, "Do you feel shame anymore?"

I'm enraged in a millisecond, and I rant about how I used to feel shame and finally just got sick of being suicidal and depressed and begging God to help me. He didn't, and I got sick of Christianity always making me feel guilty and shameful for everything. The more I talk, the sharper my words become, but it startles me when hear myself say, "I hate Christianity."

35

STRAIN MY BRAIN

Sometimes I'll be fine all day, until the sun goes down, and then I resurrect this werewolf. Tonight I eat chips out of the bag while watching a movie on my laptop at my desk. When I pause the movie to throw up, I can't get the chips out. They're too dry and they scratch my throat, which is why I usually don't eat them. They will not come up. Panic shoots through my veins because the food is not all out of my body. How much is left in my stomach, digesting, making me fat starting right now?

As I pass the mirror I study my thighs. I don't mean to look, but I do. Lillie says, even before I can consciously form a thought, "You fat, disgusting pig. You are huge. You need to go on a diet. You need to starve yourself. Just look at you. You're sickening."

As I brush my teeth, I think about being anorexic. I wonder how can I be thin and not be messed up in the head. The desire to be anorexic again never comes to fruition, because now

I know it doesn't lead to happiness. My heart doesn't want self-destruction. Maybe the truth is that I don't want to put in all the effort. More than depression, I hate structure, and that's what all eating disorders are, at the core—structured limitation, like being in a straight jacket all the time.

*

Leon will sometimes participate in my morbid defeat. I guess he thinks that if he humors me and we joke about it, then nothing bad will happen.

"Do you want me to kill you?" Leon says.

"Yes, yes, please," I say.

"Do you want me to poison you?"

"No."

"Drown you?"

"No."

"Shock?"

"No."

"Slit your throat?"

"No," I say. "Thanks for thinking of me, pal."

"Well, I'm only trying to help."

36

THE TREE'S FLEXIBILITY IS ITS STRENGTH

On my stupid, long walk to work I think about how marriage is just a clever cover-up for who I am, how none of my insecurities have been overcome. They were pushed under to bubble up again some other time. When I flip through my brain's Rolodex to find a friend I can speak honesty with, there's no one—only therapists who get paid to listen to me. I've always rewritten the truth to make it nicer and prettier and more justifiable, but it doesn't fix anything. I feel defeated, and anything to do with sexuality disgusts me, because the end result is sex.

I hate everything. Food doesn't calm me. It, too, is empty.

I stop seeing the first therapist because the second cognitive therapist specializes in eating disorders and that's a higher priority for me. But then the second therapist changes jobs and leaves me with a referral to another therapist. I haven't called yet because it's exhausting to think about telling a stranger everything from the beginning.

Upon Leon's prodding and, I suppose, my own emptiness, I finally agree to call the new therapist, whose name is Liza. At our first appointment I walk into the room and see she's tiny and blonde. *Yeah, right. There is no way she's going to be able to handle me.* So, I begin to rant about how slow my job has been at the spa.

She interrupts me, "OK, stop there."

Her words hit me like an energetic sucker punch, and my mouth half opens in amusement. I'm filled with hope.

Liza says that I desire to feel in control, so the reason I think work is hell is because I have no control over my schedule there. "You feel victimized," she says. "You sit in the staff lounge and watch other coworkers booking appointments while you have five hours of empty space on your schedule."

"Five hours of nothing, which I am not getting paid for," I say. "I want to scream, punch things, and throw rocks at the spa windows."

"Exactly," she says.

Wait. What?

"You're great at the anger emotions. You've got that covered," she says.

I do. I go back and forth between passivity and anger, shutting down in silence and blowing up, the perfectionist and the slacker.

"You've been full of a lot of things you've never wanted," she says.

My mind travels as I picture my stomach, like Santa Claus's bag stuffed full of goods like the curtains my parents bought or . . .

"What did you want?" she says.

"I wanted him to buy a goat or something . . ." I think I've started talking about having a farm.

"No, but what did you want?" she says.

I fetch an answer. ". . . to hear what I was saying?"

"Yes," she says. "You wanted to be heard."

It's funny that I don't recognize any middle ground, because I'm so busy playing take-it-all-in-like-a-zombie. Or I flip out, like I did the other day, and yell at my mom because she's told me something about Maui several times and kept talking. "Why are you still talking?"

I act out because it's my go-to coping mechanism. Restricting, binging, and puking work, to some extent, so why would I give them up? The only means I have to cope? Now, I have to find new tools, because anger only gets me so far.

"I know I'm talented in a lot of ways but I lack motivation. I have all this potential, and then the dark side of me constantly undermines everything I do."

She says, "Then you have to figure out what it is that's holding you back from your own success."

"It's because I'm lazy."

"You're not allowed to say things in the session that judge yourself and end the conversation," she says.

Whatever she asks me next makes me start talking about basketball. "When I was younger I used to be an awesome basketball player. Then I found out that the people I thought were my friends had been talking behind my back the whole year, and it destroyed me. It was the death of me."

"Can you rephrase that," she says.

"OK, it was the catalyst for my downwards spiral."

"What did you need?" she asks.

When I think hard, I don't know.

"What would you say to that little fifteen-year-old girl about it?"

"Well, of course, 'They're not your real friends. They're probably just jealous.'" As I say this, I hear my dad's voice in my head. His voice builds me up by telling me the truth, but somehow invalidates my feelings. Knowing they were jealous doesn't reach the place in my heart that's still hurt about being betrayed. "I don't know what to tell her," I say. "She's smart. She knows all this already."

"What about just saying to her, 'Yeah, that must have been extremely tough and hurtful for you.'? Then, let yourself cry, and yell, and release it instead of just pushing it down."

"So what?" I say. "How does that change anything?"

"People who deal with things sit in their feelings and feel them and get over them and move on a lot better. You pushed the feeling down and tried to pretend it didn't bother you, because you thought you were smart enough to conquer it intellectually. What lessons did that little fifteen-year-old girl get out of the situation?"

I shrug and sit there at a loss for words.

She fills in the blank. "Perhaps you learned that you can't be successful and have people like you. That you have to pick one or the other."

My eyes open a little more. I'm appalled. That's exactly what I learned. Yet, I've never in more than eleven years voiced that thought.

She draws two circles on the dry-erase board. "We have two tanks," she says, "a physical and an emotional one. You're trying to fill the emotional tank with food but the emotional tank isn't hungry for food. It wants a comforting emotional feeling. That's why food doesn't satisfy you, because you're trying to stuff it in the wrong tank. First, you need to identify the feeling you're seeking, whether it be support, clarity, or comfort. Then, figure out what you need and how you can get what you need to fill your emotional tank instead of just shoving food in it."

This should be simple, right? How am I feeling? What do I need? I see the two circles on the board. I understand what they mean, and yet, I don't identify with my feelings. Who the hell knows what I need to make myself feel better?

Instead of the depressing tape I play, she says, I need to develop a new voice that says, "OK, you're angry. What do you need?" She says that when I figure this out, even if I choose not to fulfill that need and to eat instead, at least I'll be doing it consciously.

OK, self, this is what we have to do. Go back to when we were fifteen or sixteen and figure out another way to cope instead of the eating disorder.

Liza draws on the board three circles and labels them:

Emotional mind

Rational mind

Wise mind

She says, "Emotion is like a child who's angry right now and doesn't care that he's throwing a temper tantrum in the middle of the store.

"Rational mind takes a step back to look at the whole situation and can say, 'OK, I'm angry. Why am I angry? I'm angry because I don't feel understood. I know that Leon doesn't mean to make me angry on purpose.'"

"Wise mind integrates both. It allows the anger and the rational thought and brings them together. 'OK, so what do I need from this, and how can I get it? What am I going to do with this situation?'"

I mention something about how my mom always says, "You should…" and "Don't you think?" It's just a subtle way to control me and lead my thoughts. I get incensed, because I'm so sick of being the good girl who always does what she's supposed to.

Liza says, "You can share with Leon the word/feeling connection, which goes like this: 'When you say_____, I feel _____.' Such as: 'When you say *I should,* I feel *angry.*'"

Should has always implied control to me. It makes me feel like a little kid who isn't allowed to think for herself, who's told what to feel, who's stupid and incapable of making her own decisions, who can't be trusted. *Should* leads me straight to feeling angry, furious, enraged and initiates my shutdown mechanism. I interpret the words *you should* as *I want you to be an obedient little puppet who doesn't talk back.* Basically, when people say *you should* to me it feels like they're stepping on my mind.

Liza says she could go to Paris, but she chooses to pay her mortgage instead. What I hear is, *I can't go to Paris, because I have to stay home and pay my mortgage.* I view my marriage and job as confining, because I want to travel, but I can't, because I must stay here and participate in both.

She says, "You have a lot of internalized *cant's.* Do you think you can listen to them and hear what you're telling yourself on a daily basis?"

"Maybe. So, saying *I can't* leads me to frustration, resentment, and the feeling that my life sucks?"

"Everything is a choice. Envision the choice you've made. Let's look at life as a series of choices, because it's what you choose at this point in time. There will be another point in time when you can make different choices. In controlled families there's no sense of choice or responsibility, because everything is prescribed for you."

I must have had choices, but when I looked back at my childhood, it did feel as though a lot was prescribed for me because I was a kid. Did I have choices about what I wanted? Did I ever know what I wanted? I was a good kid. I was a people pleaser. Anorexia was my good-girl way to have something to control. And then there was bulimia, my angry *Eff you!* to the world.

"I've never lived alone you know," I tell her. "I went from sharing a room with my brother to sharing a room with my college roommate to sharing a room with my husband. I constantly crave my own space, my own sense of independence. Almost daily, I teeter between wanting to be with Leon and not wanting to be with him."

"Is it that you don't want to be with Leon, or is it that you want to travel?"

Blah. No wonder I resent everything, when I see only shoulds and can'ts and negative self-talk? *I can't have what I want, damn it.*

So what is it that I want? Underneath this sucky, pissed-off attitude, what are the choices I've made that got me here? Why did I make those choices? Are those choices still consistent with what I want?

Liza says, "I'd like you to write about the things in your life, your marriage, your job, and your plans for the future. I'd like you to notice what kinds of words you use."

*

To the next session, I bring my vision board and collage of what my wise mind would look like. I tell her about this week and how I've felt stable and peaceful.

"What has worked differently?" she says.

"Well, I realized that every time I have an empty thought, it's filled immediately with the question of what I can eat. I find I eat a lot when I'm not hungry, but I've been asking myself if I'm hungry when I eat, and sometimes I am." Crazily enough, this makes me happy, and I feel like a toddler who's proud that she used the potty.

I tell Liza about my journals, how I began journaling about my marriage and Leon, but it turned into a rant about how I felt controlled as a child. "I feel this anger and irritation the more I see and realize patterns in my parents' behavior and how they affected me. The other day, Leon and my mom and I were having coffee, and I ended up being rude and mean because I blurted out, 'You already told me all this, Mom.' I don't normally talk to people like that."

She draws a triangle that represents what can happen between people or even in my relationship with an entity such as my work. Liza calls it the drama triangle. The top of the triangle is labeled V for victim, and the bottom corners are P for perpetrator, and R for rescuer.

V, Victim: hopeless or helpless, feeling like you have no power of control

P, Perpetrator: lack of responsibility

R, Rescuer: feeling obligated

The keys to avoiding the triangle are honesty and assertion through actions and words. Instead of saying, "You never listen to me," I could say, "I'm not feeling heard right now."

Liza says, "I notice that you use the words *always* and *never* a lot in conversation. These words increase the volume of your emotions."

The goal, for me, is to get off of the triangle. Even if I get myself off the triangle, there's no guarantee that I'll be able to pull the other person off. Most people don't change, even when you try completely different ways of reacting to them.

I've always joined in the dance, but I can't dance that way anymore, because it's not working. If they continue to tango, even though I'm choosing to waltz, then I need to move into acceptance mode. In acceptance mode, I'm supposed to take a personal inventory and come to a conclusion regarding how I can best take care of myself in the situation. For example, I might decide to have dinner with them only once a month. Or, I might choose to be around them for X number of hours a day. We're not the nuclear family we were when I was ten. I'm married and in my twenties; it's okay for me to set stipulations in order to be an independent adult.

Liza looks at my vision board. "It seems peaceful. It's full of nature and connection to the earth. I notice that there are hardly any people." The two images of people are far away, and we can see only the backs of their heads.

"I notice not only a lack of people, but no two people are together. Also the whole left side . . . well, actually, a majority of the board, is full of feminine energy. Feminine energy is not gender-specific, but it represents being experiential and emotional. Masculine energy, on the opposite hand, is focused on the goal and is solution-oriented. There are more words and straight lines."

"I like words," I say.

She smiles softly. "I notice that you only have a small corner of the board that's masculine." She pauses to let me review the board. "It looks like you're out of balance. You've been living an orderly life with rules and restrictions, which is all part of disordered eating, whereas what you want more of in your life is the feminine side. That could be why your whole collage consists of what you want. You're drawn towards that."

"Hmmm," is all I muster. I feel slightly off kilter.

My wise-woman collage also has a lot of symbolism of feminine energy, a lot of circles. It includes a photo of a school of fish swimming around a woman and a rainbow encircling everything on the page, all of which symbolize feminine traits.

We talk about my desire for independence. I have a hard time saying what I feel, because my default emotion is anger. Again, Liza writes out the ideal dialogue: "When you do this, I feel _____, because . . ." I rehearse the speech in my head but find myself reverting back to "I hate when . . ." or "You're so irritating."

Liza and I continue our conversation about guilt. I have a lot of resentment but haven't yet examined what I'm resentful about. Liza says I stuff and store my feelings, and repressed feelings are related to how I treat food.

She also says I focus a lot on family issues that are not mine. She asks me to try to differentiate in my mind what is my stuff and what isn't. For example, my brother's dynamic with my parents is not my issue, nor is my mom's house, which I organize even though she hasn't asked for my help. These two examples represent a plethora of duties that I take responsibility for, when they have nothing to do with me.

Liza tells me to state what I want, peacefully, over and over again like a broken record. "Yes, I appreciate that, and I want this. Yes, I appreciate that, and I want this." She says this type of communication will change my dynamic with other people, so that I won't react instinctively and be sucked into arguments. She says I'm fantastic at taking the bait and getting pulled into the fight every time.

I sigh, because I know she's right. "So, how can I give my parents feedback?"

Liza gives me a list of techniques:

1. *Talk about my feelings, not their behavior. For example, don't say, "Mom, you're so controlling," because then she'll react defensively.*

2. *Try to see my family from the outside, like a Martian looking in. Notice patterns and just observe them and try to be amused. "Isn't it interesting how excited my mom can get over sharing every detail of the dinner she cooked?"*

3. *Don't use the word* controlling *in my head. Instead, figure out the emotion. For example, "Wow, there's my mom over-loving me again. What do I want to do about it?" The word* over-loving *will replace my natural thought process that uses the words* controlling, smothering, *or* claustrophobic. *The word* controlling *turns up the volume on a thought or conversation, and my goal is to keep the volume down.*

She draws with her erasable marker a target with an outer circle, an inner circle, and a bull's-eye. She explains, "This is a dartboard. Your parents love you, so they keep throwing darts at the dartboard hoping they'll hit something. It's your job to let them know what you need, so they can hit the mark. Otherwise, they'll keep throwing darts, and you'll keep getting pissed, and everyone will be frustrated.

"It could look like this," she says. "'When you_____, I feel_____. What I need is for you to listen to me, so that I feel like I'm being heard. That would feel good.'"

It seems easy when she says it. I can't help but think it also sounds a little cheesy. I can't picture myself saying those sentences to my family in that way. But she's the therapist, so she probably knows a little bit more about relationship skills.

This week, I commit to communicating the way Liza suggests. However, when I'm in real-life situations, everything I talk about during therapy disintegrates, and I revert back to my silent or argumentative self. I like the metaphor of the target, but I'm realizing that in order to tell people where to throw the darts I should first know where the bullseye is.

"I don't think you have a problem feeling the emotions," Liza says. "You just don't have a place to put them."

Holy crap! If I have all these emotions and nowhere to put them, no wonder I feel insane. All of my emotions are constantly out in the open.

"By the way," I say, "I was having a huge amount of anxiety a couple of nights this week, for no apparent reason, and I couldn't figure out why."

"Well, anxiety wants to be fed two things: information and reassurance," Liza says. "The information aspect is where you give yourself structure and break things down into smaller pieces. You might jot things down on your calendar, so you can see your time management. If you have a free hour on Saturday, then you could say, 'What could I do with this hour?'"

I scribble frantically in my notebook trying to keep up.

"The reassurance portion might go like this, 'OK, Christen, the things on my calendar will get done. I don't know how, but they will. I trust and have faith that they will.'"

"For the first time in months it was so nice to have free time in my schedule," I tell her, "but now that the holiday break is coming to an end, I have to go back to work and school. I only have three more months of school, though. I need to just suck it up."

Liza stops me. She does that a lot, because I tend to rant, or grasp for things I can't articulate, or phrase things negatively. "Suck it up?" she says. "Notice the words you continue to use. Remember that what we do with our emotions, we do with food. You don't want to 'just suck it up,' do you?"

I don't like it when she's right, but at the same time, I do. She's like a troll hidden in a Barbie doll, and she won't let me cross the bridge unless I'm truthful. On the outside I stare blankly at her. On the inside I'm smiling. *I think she can help me get better.*

"Also," she says, "you have a habit of saying you 'have to' do something which puts you back into the drama triangle, where you become the victim. When you take on that role, you get angry."

"So, what the hell do I do, then?" This whole process is so frustrating. Everything she tells me makes sense and seems so simple when we're talking. Integrating it into my real life seems impossible.

"It's all a matter of choice," she says.

I've heard the choice speech. Everything is a choice.

"Look at what you're choosing, instead of what you're giving up. For example, by choosing to go to work, you're choosing to participate financially in your marriage and to be joyful at work."

"But what if I'm not joyful at work," I say.

"OK. If you can't be joyful about work and you're still annoyed, then stop and take a look at that annoyance. Use it. Sit with it. Sit with it, and use it to manifest thoughts about what you do want in your life."

"Sit with it" is a phrase I've heard a lot since my hospital stay. In my head, "sit with it" sounds a lot like "suck it up." Yet, "sit with it" is different. I'm not doing anything with it. It's like the Psalm, "Be still, and know that I am God."

"It's important to tell yourself a different story about work," Liza says. "Don't deny your feelings or pretend it's a Pollyanna world. However, how much you suffer depends on what you tell yourself."

I suffer a lot. I must be telling myself the wrong things.

My vision board indicates I'm seeking feminine energy, which means that I don't spend a lot of time nurturing my femininity. If my vision board is mostly feminine, it means I hold too much masculine energy, exemplified in my anorexia, perfectionism, and performance anxiety. The imbalance reveals itself in my shoulds and have-tos, because I am the ruthless taskmaster. Liza says it's interesting how she remembers me saying I wanted nothing to do with anything feminine, yet that is what shows up all over my vision board.

Fuck.

Liza points out that when I was younger, I never had the freedom to decide how I felt, because I was told, or my needs were met before I realized I needed anything. I feel strange about this. The insight is confusing to me, because my parents were awesome, yet they hindered me. One of Angelina Jolie's tattoos says, "What nourishes me also destroys me."

"What are things that I could say that acknowledge my parents' good intentions and reinforce that I can take care of myself?"

"Good question," she says. "Can you think of some things you could say to your parents?"

My mind is a totally blank slate. "It's like I'm treading into unknown territory. I don't even know how to say hello in this new language."

"OK," she says, "I'll give you some examples. Let's say your parents keep asking you questions about your life, because they love you. You could respond with, 'I appreciate your concern. I appreciate that you want to help, but it's important to me that I do this on my own.' Or you could say, 'I appreciate you trying to support me, but that doesn't validate my feelings. What I need right now is for you to allow me to feel____ right now and have that be OK and not try to fix it.' Or you could tell them something as simple as, 'I appreciate your concern, but I'm OK.'"

Her last example reminds me of my infamous childhood retort, "I can do it myself." The truth is that I can't do it by myself. If I were able, I wouldn't be in therapy getting instructions on how to talk with my own parents.

37

THE VOICES IN MY HEAD

Lately, Lillie talks to me all the time, except when I'm watching the Simpsons, which I watch at night after the sun goes down. I named her so I could separate the good in me from the bad in her. She's suffocating, but she's so pretty and sly that I keep letting her back in. She's the master of tricks. In the end, I always need enough food to feed her and hope that she'll leave me alone. But I don't know who I'd be if she were gone.

A new voice is showing up in my head lately. It's Liza's. It's the things I've heard her say in therapy. Fragments of our conversations replay, and I can use her voice to talk to Lillie. I'm sick of Lillie's lies, and I'm sick of her friendship that makes me feel as though I'm never good enough.

When I was in the hospital, they told us, "The eating disorder is not your friend. It is trying to kill you. And if it wins, you will die." On one of our group outings, I bought a plaster skull as a reminder. After I left the hospital, it hung out on my bookshelf, then in the fish tank, and now in the corner of the shower I share with my husband.

When I unpacked my suitcase after coming home from the hospital, Leon picked the skull up and arched his eyebrow. "You're so morbid," he said, giving his head a little shake and wondering why I hadn't managed to grow up and be normal.

Since the day I bought the skull, I've kept it in view to scare me, but it didn't work. Lillie mocks, "The way you eat isn't going to kill you. Look how long you've been doing it."

My voice sometimes agrees. *My tests have turned up normal. I'm not half as bad as the girls in the hospital. I can eat and have a conversation. When I was anorexic, I ate three meals a day. I ate good food before the bad, so I didn't throw up stomach acid, and I drank water afterwards. I'm nowhere near as bad.*

Shit. That sounds a lot like Lillie's voice. She waves at me in the distance as I realize the truth, my truth, that this whole ordeal has killed me spiritually, withered me one poison spoonful at a time until my rainbow soul is drained of color and resembles the moldy white skull in our shower.

What's the point of secrets? Do they protect or destroy? Jesus was an advocate of truth, no matter how uncomfortable. He was also an advocate of compassion. In high school, we studied Emily Dickinson, whose poetry said, "Tell all the truth but tell it slant." Jesus might have said, "Tell all the truth but season it with compassion."

We're taught that friends keep secrets. But what if those secrets hurt? The things Lillie told me, I've accepted as absolute truth: *I'm lazy. No one likes me. I'm weak. If I were thinner, I would have more power and confidence, and people would respect me. Then I would be someone. Then I could relax. Then I would be happy.*

Without question, I listened like a good little girl and believed everything she fed me. I believed that God was disappointed in me, that I could never make Him proud, that He was growing sick of my broken promises, and that He had left me to struggle on my own because I wasn't good enough.

*

Liza tells me the language we use is powerful. I'm setting myself up for depression with the language I use to talk to myself. "Unhook from rebelling," she says.

Anytime I tell myself I *have to* do something, I don't just rebel, I *Fuck you!* rebel.

"It's not that you have to do something," she says, "but that you choose to. If you switch the words, you can no longer rebel, because there's no one to rebel against."

Next, we talk about my wants. What are the little things that I can do in my little bit of free time? How can I dangle little carrots daily instead of waiting for the big carrot at the end?

It's a good chance to practice my self-soothing and self-care. I don't want to go to work, but I'm going to:

Wear some clothes that I like

Play a CD I enjoy

Liza says it's the small pleasures that add joy to our lives.

Then, we talk about food journaling and how it marks the journey of recovery. When I get full, it's a trigger for my disorder. Since I moved back to Hawai'i, I've been able to cope during the day by eating snacks or fruit, so I don't get too full, triggered, or distracted from my tasks. I bide my time until dinner, when I have a big meal. When I was younger, the night used to make me feel alive, but now it traps me like a caged animal, and I creep around my house, antsy and looking for a binge. Something about darkness calls Lillie out to play. In the darkness, she's a hunter, and nothing distracts her from the food she stalks. In the darkness, she no longer deprives herself of all the food she can eat and throw up.

Liza writes some numbers on her dry-erase board. "On a scale of one to ten, number one is starving. Five is neutral. Ten is purge. When you're at a three, that means it's time to eat, and when you're at a seven or eight is when you could choose to stop eating."

The two-bite technique: eat two bites and put down the fork and check my stomach's fullness on a scale of one to ten. In theory, it sounds like a great idea, but my body has become so detached from what's normal that I have no concept of what my body feels from one to ten. I'm throwing numbers out just to appease her.

"I don't know. Four? I can't remember the last time I felt physically hungry when I ate. I don't remember the normal feeling of fullness, because anytime I feel full, I stop it by throwing up." *Out you go, food. Out you go, feeling of being full.*

I watch people push back their plates and smile as they say, "I'm so full." They're happy about that? Being full is a horrible feeling. I want to get rid of it immediately. Like *Tell Tale Heart,* it's under the floorboard beating *Out,*

out, out, out, out, out, out, slowly driving me insane. It's the same anxious compulsion I remember feeling with anorexia, when my mind wouldn't stop its rant unless I complied and went running to burn calories. With a peaceful smile or calm wave, I'd meander across campus, while inside everything felt constricted. *Hurry hurry run run run run run run run run. Run run run. Out out out.* I always complied. The squeaky wheel gets the oil. The incessant voice gets appeased.

Liza is telling me, "What we do with emotions, we do with food."

Huh?

I polarize my emotions. For me, there is only black and white, no gray middle ground. Thus, I polarize my behavior with food: all or nothing, good or bad, anorexic or bulimic. "It seems that you eat only one real meal a day," she says.

"Well, yes. I like one big meal, because that way I don't have to be full for long at night. I know that breakfast is supposed to be the most important meal of the day, but if I start out full first thing in the morning, then I binge and purge all day long. It's so much more manageable to deal with just the evening hours instead of the entire day."

She stares at me, as if gathering the words to delicately tell me how the way I think is messed up. "The projections," she says, "are your internal have-tos and what you project that others are making you do."

This is true. When I told my dad I didn't want to go back to school, he gave me the, "You can't drop the ball now" deal. I realize now that the harsh masculine voice I use to talk to myself is my dad's voice. But I don't know how to talk to myself differently. I've been doing it for so long.

"Let's try something," Liza suggests. "Let's rewrite a different story about school in a voice that you can believe. Let's put in the comforting pieces and the rewards, so that the process isn't as painful. The words and the language you use cause you to suffer more. The word *choose* places the power with you. The words *I want to* do the same. The words *have to, need to, should, must* are clearly not helpful. The masculine voice says, 'OK, so you're going to go to school.' This voice is linear and goal-oriented, focused on the factual statement. The feminine voice says, 'OK, so what would help you suffer less?'"

The problem with little rewards on a list is that I don't make a habit of bestowing them. Despite the fact that I make one almost every day, lists have never worked for me. I once wrote a list of at least fifty things I could do instead of throw up. None of them worked. I could do all fifty of them and still want to throw up, still think about throwing up the whole time I was doing all fifty of them. I can be two different people at the same time. I can collage and not be present. I can go through the motions, but for whom? The list of rewards is its own problem, too, because deep down I don't think I'm worth rewarding. I have a good life compared to so many people. What a huge baby I am complaining about it. What the hell is wrong with me?

I hear Liza's voice in my head. "Well, that's not your reality. Your reality is your life."

I feel guilty for suffering, because I've deemed my suffering unworthy compared to other people who have real problems. But how is throwing up every day not a big problem? How have I justified this to myself for so long?

*

After I keep food down for a few days, my side begins to ache. Screw what Liza says about patience! I do the Master Cleanse. On the second day of the juice fast, I sit exhausted and negative on Liza's couch. I know she's frowning about my decision, but I don't know what else to do to make the pain stop.

I believe certain things are healthy, like eating vegan and raw and fasting occasionally, but my beliefs go against what I actually want, which is to eat cookies and shave ice and gobble lots and lots of food. Neither extreme brings me happiness.

Liza says I could find a happy medium in between, like 80% of what I know is good food and 20% of what I want. Coincidentally, that's the raw foods diet equation: 80% raw, 20% cooked. I'm coming to realize that perhaps raw is not the right choice, because it's dangerous for me, according to Asian medicine. My acupuncturist told me she used to believe in eating raw, but she ended up getting sick. She now believes in balance.

Today, my homework is to write out my beliefs about food and the rules that guide my eating and then examine them and decide which ones are true and which are false. For example, my knee pain prevents me from running. I could swim or do yoga, but my mind immediately jumps to the conclusion, *Well, I can't run. Screw it. I'm going to do nothing.*

"Your thinking is permanent and negative." Liza says.

I don't know what to say to that. It sounds destructive when I hear her say it. Permanent. Negative. I sit there and furrow my brow, which I assume she has come to recognize as meaning I get what she's saying, but I'm at a loss as to how to move forward differently.

"You could say, 'Right now running hurts. Right now I'm choosing to swim. I'm not sure about tomorrow, but right now this is what I'm choosing.' This way of talking to yourself makes the choice transient. 'Right now.' Notice the transient nature."

I do notice. My body relaxes. How is it that I never thought I had options? Why did I just focus on my injured knee and say, *Screw it?* How did I condition my brain to see no other pathways or choices?

She ends therapy with a kicker, "What makes you happy besides food?"

"Happy? What's that? I like reading, being in nature, listening to music. But happy? I feel happy when I'm free. I can't remember the last time I felt free."

38

A BALANCING OF HEAD AND HEART

Even when Leon and I are laughing, my mind is running in multiple parallel lanes like the separate lanes around a track. I'm the runner, and I'm in all the lanes. We're laughing and watching TV, and although I'm there on the bed with him, my mind is in the kitchen, in the bathroom, at the grocery store, going through the cabinets, scanning the freezer, watching the clock. My mind is exhausted from all the exercise.

In Liza's office, I ramble about work, sinking into a deep black hole. I can almost see the heaviness and hear the muck. "All my choices are false choices," I tell her. "It's like I'm faking, but the positive side is that it's all just a joke and I'm fooling myself. It's like I'm trying to trick myself but part of me is too smart for tricks."

"Your list," she says, after I've read to her the seventeen rules that govern my eating, "is negative and rigid and filled with absolutes, typical of an anorexic mindset."

"I just want peace. I want one day that I don't have to fight myself and hate myself."

"OK, let's take on one belief you have, say the one about eating desserts. What are you telling yourself when you eat desserts? What's going on in your head? Let's say you eat a cookie."

Rules and absolutes go through my mind. This conversation makes me want five cookies. "I mean, I know cookies aren't good for me, but I like them, and I still want to eat them."

Sensing my rigidity, she responds, "The way you write is polarized and rigid."

No kidding.

"You write negative thoughts as though they are absolute truths." She asks me to rewrite my list. "Look it over again and consider it for rigidity. Try to allow some wiggle room, to consider what's emotionally good for you. Ask yourself questions. 'Can I live this way? Is it healthy for me?' Come up with some new ways of thinking."

I deal with food the same way I deal with everything. I either embrace life with no rules or I allow only the rigid structure of my own design.

Work is: I have to. I don't want to. Because I see work as the enemy, controlling me and forcing me to be structured, I pout. I treat food the same way. I deprive myself or indulge to the point of disgust. I let myself be walked on, or I lash out.

How can I be more in balance, so I feel like I'm a willing participant and not just a pawn? Where is the happy medium—that balance between absolute structure and chaotic free fall? It's a place somewhere between black and white, where I happily make the right choice to live in the rainbow of color and life. Rainbows, I was told as a child, are God's promise that He'll never again send a flood to destroy the earth.

39

THE MESSAGE PAIN GIVES US

Since I moved back to Hawai'i, I work at a spa where I make half the money I made in California for the same work. I decide to enroll in massage school to gain a skill that I can barter without the need for equipment. I go from working at the spa all day to class at night and get home around ten o'clock. It's exhausting but interesting.

In *lomi lomi* massage class we learn how memories are stored in the body, how they are locked with a secret combination, and we can go years without accessing them. Then, one day someone is massaging your hip and the numbers align, the lock opens, and you begin to cry. Someone stretches your neck a certain way and you think of your mom or your dad, and a memory becomes so real you feel it as though you're experiencing it again.

An anorexic person cuts her senses off at the neck to remove all connection to the body. The bulimic person can't handle the overwhelming feelings. The solutions are starving it out or throwing it up, but either way the result is emptiness. For most of my life I have overridden my body—pushed my intellect, lived in my thoughts, and disconnected from my body.

The phantom side pain brings my focus to my physical self. Pain is my new adversary, and, yes, I do fear it.

Liza says that all pain gives us a clear and simple message. "What if you become friends with it?" she asks me.

My heart quivers and I crinkle my face. *Become friends with my nemesis?*

The thing that torments me? It's like asking Superman to become friends with Lex Luthor.

"What if you do?" she says. "Let's just say that the pain will not go away. What if the positive choice to move forward is to befriend your enemy? What if you said, 'OK, pain, you and I are going to be friends, so let's get to know each other. What is it that you want me to know?'"

"My decision to throw up is largely based on the memory of my side pain," I say, "and the fear that if I keep all my food down, the pain will return, and I'll be helpless."

The black leather couch always seems like a huge time machine that allows me to shuffle through my memories at lighting speed. *I should be smarter than this and be over this already. I will not cry during this session.*

I hate crying in front of other people, but I became friends with a girl named Di in massage school, and I can cry with her. She's the first friend outside the hospital I've told the whole truth about my eating disorder. I felt more comfortable with her because she was a raw foodist. She didn't understand everything about the disorder, but she didn't look at me as though I were a freak or give me that fearful, blank stare.

Di asked me questions, and I told her everything. Afterwards, I worried whether she would treat me differently the next time I saw her. And she did: we became closer.

Liza draws a wave on the dry-erase board. "If your pain is like this wave, when it begins to swell with anger, annoyance, and anxiety it produces a fight-or-flight reaction."

In surfing, the drop is what caused me to chicken out of the wave. The same terror grips me when I'm full, when my stomach is distended, when all the memories of side pain, not being able to go to the bathroom, dizzy spells, and hopelessness rush back. I eat the food, but I don't like the view of the drop. I lean over the toilet and turn my stomach like a wave until it all comes pouring out.

"If the emotional wave is going to peak at two feet high," Liza explains, "you stop the wave at one foot by throwing up. You never give it a chance to calm down again."

"Well, yeah," I say, "I cut it off because I'm terrified it will get bigger and bigger and crush me."

"But you forget that waves go up and down," she says, simulating the motion with the marker. "The up doesn't last forever. Neither does the down. Out of fear, you're not riding the wave. You're emptying your stomach before you give yourself a chance to make peace with the terror."

She draws on the board the cycle of feelings feeding thoughts, thoughts feeding behavior, and then the behavior feeding the feelings over and over.

"Your questions, your 'what if's,' project you into a future you don't know. If you keep thinking of all the possibilities, yet you don't want to do anything because the idea becomes so overwhelming, then you can't move."

"So what can I do?"

"What if you told yourself a different story about the pain? What does it look like? Can you draw it?"

"It's like a black fuzzy ball with sharp spikes slicing through my colon."

"Let's make a different picture of that pain," she says. "Let's see if we can move it through your body without the spikes digging in."

Through the course of therapy I've become aware that there's a metaphorical toolbox full of techniques I can develop to facilitate growth and healing. As Liza says, I used to go to the bakery for a hammer and then get mad because all they had was bread. Of course they had loaves of bread. I went to the bakery, not the hardware store. I used to go to people who weren't good listeners, and I expected to be heard but became hurt and angry because I didn't feel validated.

"Trying to white-knuckle it through the pain is a harder way," she says. "Put that stick in the spokes of the bicycle wheel. Fear is keeping you in the vicious cycle. Getting out is a leap of faith. You're going to have to trust."

How can I trust myself when I don't trust myself?

My plan is similar to practicing a fire drill in case there's a fire. I'll eat just what I can handle and then self-soothe and ride it out. Practice with my toolkit. Visualize the pain. It's not anchored in my side. It has no spikes.

But memories are strong, and they tend to override the present plan. Like heavy duty magnets, they attract me to another time, when I was someone else.

How can I trust myself when I don't trust myself?

40

CAN YOU KILL THE GHOSTS?

I am a bulimic walking around with the remnants of an anorexic mind. The question is plaguing me: do you ever really recover?

A stanza from an Ani DiFranco song[1] comes to mind.

They say that an alcoholic is always an alcoholic
Even if he's dry as my lips for years.
Even if he's stranded on a small desert island
With no place in two thousand miles to buy beer.
And I wonder is he different;
Is he different, has he changed what he's about?
Or is he just a liar with nothing to lie about?

"A liar with nothing to lie about." Will I still think about food most of the day, whether I eat it or not? Will I be able to look in the mirror and not hear my mind screaming obscenities or whispering all the ways it can improve me? Will I be able to look at myself in the mirror and say, "I'm happy"? Will it be the truth? Or is this just like being an alcoholic with no alcohol around?

Liza tells me that she believes I can put it all behind me, but at the same time, recovery is an up-and-down process, not just an inclining straight line.

---

[1] Ani Difranco, "Fuel," by Ani Difranco, In *Little Plastic Castle*, Righteous Babe, 1998, compact disk.

Even though I may be exhibiting the same behavior, it doesn't mean I'm mentally in the same place. She says, "Trust yourself to make the best choices you know how to make. Keep moving. There is strength in that."

41

NIGHT IS WHEN THE DARKNESS CALLS

Choice. I don't know to what to do with it. In order to recover, I must want something more than the anorexia or bulimia.

This time, when I watch *American Beauty* the plastic bag scene that usually has me crying like a baby doesn't affect me at all. What was so powerful this time? The final scene, when Lester talks to Angela in the kitchen, and he asks her about his daughter. He says, "Is she happy?" and Angela smirks and replies, "She's really happy . . . She thinks she's in love." A little smile spreads across Lester's face as though his life is complete and he can now be at peace. A few seconds later, he's dead.

I think of my dad's question floating there like a birthday balloon, "Are you happy?" It's what every parent wants for his kid: happiness. He can depart in peace with a little smile on his face, the one that says, "I can go now. She's going to be okay."

*

Forbidding certain foods, according to Liza, is why I eat them and throw them up. Because they are forbidden, I can get rid of them. Her solution is more protein, more carbs, or more nutrient-dense food, because it doesn't take much to get full. "You might have to choose what you eat carefully."

Somehow this sounds like a threat, as if I'm teetering on the edge and the weight of one little spoonful will make me fall.

"What you're choosing to do with food cannot work right now," Liza says. "At least, not right now."

I sink into the cold black leather couch with the silence of defeat. *I can't do what I believe in, because I'm not normal.*

"You're still in the eating disorder, and we have to deal with what *is*. Do you agree with that?" She speaks slowly, her voice calm and steady, as if a piece of yarn tied loosely to my wrist could keep me from falling. But it does. It's enough to make me believe I am tethered, to keep me attentive.

"I suggest you write after you eat. Write about what you feel at night. Write about why you feel trapped."

During the day around my house, birds sing relentlessly, as though they're trying to tell me why I do unhealthy things. They watch me with their beady eyes, ruffle their feathers, and walk like an Egyptian across the back steps. When night comes, I look out the window at the little bird that sleeps with his eyes closed and his mouth snapped shut. All the secrets of his song remain trapped behind the slight curve of his beak.

I haven't said a word. Liza has been sitting quietly in her chair, watching. "What's going on for you?" she asks.

How do I begin to explain how my mind throws me down several rabbit holes at once? In thirty seconds, entire conversations occur. No solutions, just the voices prodding and poking.

"At night, something shifts," I say. "It's like I'm boxed in, like my mind gets claustrophobic. I want to do so many things. I have all these fantastic ideas, and then I just get lazy and sabotage myself. Then I turn on the TV and eat. I hate myself for that."

42

IT'S ALL SUCH STRANGE VIOLENCE

Strange and violent dreams haunt me. In them, I die when a fuzzy black ball with sharp spikes explodes in my belly. When I wake up, I feel like Lillie's been feeding me spiky black seeds in my sleep and cultivating them by wearing me down. In the real world, I keep my rage at bay by playing the nice girl, but I'm afraid I'm not so nice on the inside anymore. What if one day Lillie wins? What if the poison seeds she's sown take over, and one morning I wake up, and she replaces me and carries on as the one in control?

*

I tell Liza everything—verbally throwing up all over her office. She sits in her chair, barely moving as I spew everything, not knowing what's important. I share how being around my brother and his girlfriend pains me. The lightness about them, their confidence and freedom strike me like sunshine hitting my eyes after I've been in a dark cave. I look at my brother's girlfriend, who seems self-aware and self-confident. I shy away from her, because being close to her makes me feel less than perfect and reminds me how far I am from becoming the person I want to be. I find opportunities to drop out of the conversation.

I've spent many years making a home for this disease, feeding it like a monster by doing what it wants, in the hope that it will stay contained. I've been feeding a monster whose one goal is to kill me, and the more I feed it, the stronger it becomes. "You will never be free. You will never be normal.

You're worthless. You're so far from your goal. You don't even know who you are. You're fat. You're lazy. You're pathetic and worthless. I know you hear the words I say, and I am never going away."

Liza looks me straight in the eye, "You have to stay on the journey. Even though you think you're going backwards, you are not in the same place."

I shrug. I don't believe her. I still binge and purge. I still can't stop it. "And the difference is?"

"For example, the cycles seem to have lost a lot of their power. They're not an absolute compulsion like they used to be for you in California. You do have a desire to stop, and you have a lot of awareness."

"Well, then, if I'm smart, which I know I am, and I'm aware of all this, then why can't I just stop?" I sound desperate. My eyes are down. I'm scribbling something on my notepad.

Her soft voice is like a feather full of lightning. "Well, you don't yet trust that you have another skill that will work. You've been using this one tool in your toolbox for so long that it's become the only one you trust. It's the one you reach for every single time. Recovery," she says, "is when you are free from binging and purging. When you can accept your body most of the time. When, most of the days, you don't obsess about food."

I stop writing and stare straight at her. "That's just not good enough for me. To me, that's just like being an addict without using the drug."

"I don't think about it in that way," she says. "An alcoholic is addicted to the product, to the actual alcohol." She lets me mentally agree with this. "You're not addicted to food," she says. "You're addicted to the process of numbing out." She stays silent and watches as my brain rants quietly inside my head.

"It's a process," Liza interrupts my rant, "and who you are going to be afterwards is someone who has integrated the eating disorder into her life. Look at how far you've come already. Look at all the changes in you that support the end of the eating disorder."

Liza has told me that to purge is the biggest *Fuck you!* there is. "If you're going to throw up, at least know why you're doing it. Write, because there's something under that. When you say, 'My food just doesn't digest well,' there's something else behind that thought. And that something else is the key to not throwing up."

"OK. So, when I throw up, there are a few possibilities. Am I being clear in my communication? Am I being resentful? Am I being indirect? Sometimes I wonder if there is a 'better,' a space where I'll be free from all of this."

"Better isn't a destination," she tells me. "Better is a process. It's ongoing. It never ends. You get there, and when you're there, you keep going."

43

THE SCARS

Getting better requires commitment, but because I'm used to breaking promises I don't trust myself. I don't want to let anyone down, because that reinforces I'm a liar. Sometimes I think that if I'm going to hate myself either way, I might as well give up and let Lillie win.

A little mockingbird saunters across the concrete with the cocky swagger of a miniature tyrannosaurus.

My mind is powerful. I just have to find a way to focus on the right things. I can't let Lillie win. She's the one who limits me. She puts me in boxes and cages that have locks without keys. She brainwashes me to hate myself and be a negative person. And because Lillie is me, who needs Satan? I do his bidding while he reclines on the couch with his cocky grin and I beat myself in the corner.

Liza tells me I'm intelligent and articulate, and when I get into my negative space, it's easy for me to rationalize what I'm doing. "You're also determined," she says, "which can be detrimental. You're able to convince yourself of things, so you can still feel in control."

Like the fact that throwing up is a fantastic idea, and it will solve my problems.

"When your mind is spinning, you need peace, because you're not thinking clearly enough to find a good solution. I suggest you sit on the couch and focus on breathing."

I can't help but stare as though we're having two different conversations.

"If you were going to spend ten minutes eating," she says, "why not spend it breathing?" *Um, hello! So many reasons. What does breathing give me? It's like offering a fish air when all it craves is water.*

My emotional mind spins and spins, while my wise mind needs some time to say, "OK, what am I going to do to help myself?" My wise mind seeks the bigger picture, but I keep throwing it off with my spinning. I hear Liza's voice in my head, *"When the irritation rises, jam a stick in the spokes of the wheel, so you stop."*

"You need to trust that you are going to be okay," Liza tells me.

I look away, as if the words sting. Each remission of my eating disorder has been followed by an even deeper pit of binging and purging. Tears run towards the floor and I don't even bother to wipe them away. I do not trust that Lillie will ever go away.

"You *need* to trust that you are going to be okay," she says.

44

THE ONLY ONE THAT TALKS

At a family gathering, a little boy sees me and disappears into the house, returning with his DVD of *Pirates of the Caribbean*. He points to the picture of Keira Knightly and back to me, saying I look like her. I think this is a compliment; people think she's pretty. *What does a little boy know, though?* Just then, the boy's mom comes home from work, strolls up to the porch, and gives me an emphatic hug. "You look good. Like you got a little more meat on your bones."

She says this as a genuine compliment. The sound part of my brain knows this is good. The unhealthy part says, *What?* The unhealthy part sounds the alarm, making me twinge and want to vomit. I let out a laugh and say, "Thanks," because I don't know what else to say.

"The last time she saw you, you were skinnier," Lillie whispers.

Shut up, I say confused. *I thought I looked skinny today. Is that not true? What if I just think I'm skinny when I'm fat? What if I can't even tell the difference anymore?* My hands grip my pockets as if trying to keep me rational, to keep my mind from running the distance.

I feel better when people tell me how skinny I look, and Lillie says, "Yes. Great job. You won. You succeeded. You stand out. You're unique." But the truth is that being skinny doesn't make me unique. It lumps me with a group of other people with the same distorted way of thinking the same thing. How special is that?

45

THE THINGS WE DO INSTEAD

"I think you underestimate your ability to deal with your uncomfortable feelings," Liza tells me. I sit there thinking she's full of lies.

Liza and I have been talking for a few months now. When she leans back in her chair and sighs, she tells me I have enough information, that I am a smart woman, that I am now at a point in my recovery where I actually have to pull out my tools and commit to getting better.

The word *commitment* makes me cringe, because I am a liar. I have uttered hundreds of promises that I've broken within minutes. *Commitment* is a scary word, because it threatens the liar in me and dangles rigidity before my eyes.

"You must commit," Lillie smiles. "You must do this all perfectly, or else you're an utter failure."

The problem is none of my tools work. Over the years, I've made hundreds of lists of things to do and ways to self-soothe, which are only momentary distractions. I've tried wearing tangible reminders like jewelry, statements like "I believe," coloring, going for walks, telling myself the reasons I would die if I didn't stop. Nothing. Nothing. Nothing works. Nothing even remotely comes close.

They say the eating disorder serves some purpose, otherwise I would not have chosen it. If the real threat of sudden death isn't enough to scare me, then there's something I'm protecting, that I hold onto, in spite of the possibility that my eating disorder will kill me.

"What is going to help you then?" Liza asks. Then she sits there for at least a minute in silence.

"This whole time, I've let other people tell me what I should do. They told me that I should make lists, so I did, even when the lists didn't work. Ever."

"Think about a scenario in the future, then," Liza says.

An image immediately comes to mind. I'm in Italy. I'm traveling. I'm in a restaurant with a group of my friends sitting around a table. The lights exude a soft candle-like glow in the cozy space between the dark outside and the deep red of our wine glasses. The round table is covered with an array of food. We sit together, laughing. I'm in the moment, in the laughter, in the conversation, enjoying the food and the people. I don't know where the bathroom is or how strongly the toilet flushes. I don't know how much or what everyone else has eaten, because I haven't been monitoring the food. The people fill me—my friends, their words, their smiles—and I'm holding my glass of wine and eating bites of food between the words of conversation. And I'm glowing with the electric energy of what it feels like to be free and happy.

This is what I'll hold. This will be my only tool, because it's the only tool that will work, because I've decided not to self-soothe, or try to distract myself in the moment, but instead to push my mind into a future I can create with decisions I make today.

Pep talk: *OK, if you want to get there, to your restaurant in Italy, it starts today. It starts now. Practice now. You want to hold the power, so do it. This is completely your choice.*

46

RISKING

This week, I'm hopeful as I tell Liza about my progress. This week, I've kept all the food down.

"Yes," she says, "you have taken some scary risks by keeping food down."

I am good. It's been terrifying, when the fullness sets in, to allow the food to remain in my stomach, allow myself to be full, force myself to stay that way. I hope that I can do it—that I will one day sit in that restaurant in Italy and feel free.

This week, I've been watching people eat at work. I see what they bring in their little plastic containers and to-go boxes: rice, meat, pasta. I would never put in my mouth 99% of what my coworkers eat, and yet they eat this stuff every day, and none of them are blowing up like blimps. Not all of them are exactly thin, but they're not gaining weight. In fact, they're staying the same size in spite of the crap they're putting into their mouths on a daily basis.

Why haven't I noticed this before? If other people eat horrible food and don't get fat, then I should be able to be full and not get fat as well. *The full-equals-fat equation, is not true.* I'm feeling hopeful.

Earlier this week, I made curtains for my house. It's symbolic, because this week I made such huge progress with my eating. The curtains symbolize finally taking control of my life.

My mom walked through the door and noticed them immediately. "Oh," she said, "I like your curtains. You made them. How cool." And she smiled.

All the things I thought my mom might say, she didn't. In fact, she shocked me with her peaceful, positive response.

I was expecting something like, "Oh, you didn't like the other curtains anymore?" or "Why did you take them down?" or the guilt trip, "It's your house you can do whatever you want."

Perhaps this whole time I've anticipated their hypothetical preexisting negative reactions without giving them a chance to prove otherwise. I notice how something as simple as a response to my new curtains can propel me further towards my recovery.

Since I'm taking emotional risks, now that I'm consciously not throwing up, it helps to have the simple motivation of my mom's response validating that I can be the person I want to be. I've begun to draw pictures of this person. She has multicolored hair and lives in the rainbow between the extremes of black and white.

47

WHAT I KNOW

For the first time since I was fifteen, I am consciously creating the person I want to be. Everything is being examined as I put myself together like a puzzle, trying to figure out what fits.

Leon keeps talking about defining things.

At this stage, non-negotiables don't exist. I can say that I'm never going to throw up, again until I do, and then I become a liar. I'm sick of being a liar; therefore, I'm careful not to define anything concretely just yet.

Leon says that in our marriage we should have non-negotiables, because otherwise we can be made to consider other things. What I think he means is other people. This makes logical sense, except that right now I don't want to be defined or boxed in by anything that tells me who I am or who I should be.

*

Leon books a trip to the outer island for a couple days so we can vacation together.

For the first time since high school, I go through an entire vacation without throwing up once and without Lillie harassing me about it. It's the first time my mind has felt free since I was fifteen. I'm not consumed with thoughts of food all day.

I examine myself and find a strange, new person who is borrowing my body and my mind, who is oddly healthy and tells me good things I'm not used to hearing. I stare at her as if she grew from the seeds of some shriveled plant I'd stopped watering long ago.

The world seems to have morphed overnight from a scary place I can't trust, where I was just one cashew away from a binge and purge, to this strange world of choices where I define myself by the choices I've made or am making.

48

THE BLACK AND WHITE WAYS I VIEW THE WORLD

During the eleven years I've had my eating disorder, I've had a lot to say, but when I was shy, when I feared rejection, when I didn't trust myself, I was silent. Recovery is a process of acquiring: knowledge, experience, positive tools, a voice. It's also a process of shedding: destructive patterns, Lillie. It's not easy. That's why I must be brutally honest. If I can't be honest with myself, I won't recover. Period.

Did the hospital magically fix me like I thought it was going to? No. But it did provide me with a seed of hope for the possibility of getting better. Since my hospital stay, I've been digging for the truth below the statement, "I have an eating disorder because I don't want to be fat."

I've been walking 'round and 'round the labyrinth towards the center, wherein lies the scroll of wisdom. In my hands, it's warm and as light as a feather. My fingers tremble as I break the seal. Words curl along the page, the color of blood. "Christen, you're scared of being fat. It's why you don't leap. You have enough information. You must apply it. You must eat and keep the food down. You must leap in faith, and I will catch you."

I picture myself as little girl. I'm standing at the edge of a cliff. I'm afraid to move because I might fall. My back begins to itch, and I realize I'm growing tiny wings.

49

THE NEW REALITY OF MY LIFE

Two weeks and counting: no binging or throwing up. This is going to be my life—keeping all the food down. It's the scariest thing I've ever had to do. My mind flies into panic mode and stages a protest, frantically pacing through my skull, wide-eyed, waving streamers, and shouting violently.

It's hard to hate Lillie. Recovery involves letting go of her alluring voice and the familiar bruises of her kisses, like purple flowers blossoming against my mouth. She calls to me like a siren with her long, jet-black hair. The plummy fullness of her lips mesmerizes me. She's always wanted me. Letting her go is like a long, slow-motion French kiss. Craving her still, I peel myself away and pant, inches from her lips, while her touch smolders under my skin like fire.

The taste of plums lingers on my tongue as I struggle to accept my victory. As destructive as Lillie was, I have the unsteady feeling that I've lost her.

50

A QUEST FOR THIS BODY

A bag of sugar. A bag of flour. A fully grown Chihuahua. A pair of work boots. A half-gallon of paint. Each of these items weighs five pounds. Five pounds. Roughly five pounds is the reason I was willing to risk sudden death.

How much do I want to be free?

Issues with body image are the first to creep in at the start of the eating disorder and the last to be conquered during recovery. I'm terrified to face the mirror on the wall that silently judges me. *What if I get fat? What if my digestive system shuts down again, like it did in Germany? What if I'm in pain every day? What if I want to die?*

Anger and frustration mask the fact that I'm scared. I must convince myself constantly that I cannot, *I will not*, go back. *If I want to get better I must step off the cliff.*

Skinny is still the yardstick I use to compare myself to others. *At least I'm skinnier. I've won.* But what have I won? Skinny never equaled joy.

Being recovered means I won't be able to rely on being skinny to make me feel worthy. I'll have to be more than my looks. I'll have to excel in my potential instead of pushing it down. I'll have to embrace myself as more than one-dimensional. I can't change anything from here on without self-love.

51

OUT OF LOVE

I've been told that, as I recover and get to know myself, my relationships with those closest to me will change. Most people don't end up staying with the partners they were with when they had their eating disorders. The recovered eating-disordered person is very different. She develops her own voice. Sometimes, it turns out, her partner liked her better when her voice wasn't as strong.

As my eating becomes more stable, I find the rest of me zooming all over the place like a particle bomb exploding in all directions. Leon doesn't know what to do with me, and I can sense that he's getting anxious about my new whims. My new world-travel plans seem to be a reality waiting at my fingertips except for one thing: him. In my mind, he's the tether that keeps me from being able to leap into the great big world. Lillie held me down, but now that I'm starting to wriggle free, I realize that my marriage feels like another choker chain.

When we said our marriage vows, we wanted to be married. This is what we agreed to. When Leon said his vows, he meant them. When I said them . . . It's not that I didn't mean them, but what I think I meant was, "You make me so happy, and I want to be with you." He was committed to forever. I was desperately grasping at happiness.

I've changed our marriage by voicing things that for six and a half years have not been part of our reality, things like, "Hey, Leon, I want to travel to

Bali with Di for a month or two . . . I want to go to India and study at an ashram." He gives me the frowny stare and we have huge arguments. He fights to preserve our marriage, which he is certain my traveling will destroy. I demand absolute freedom and call him rigid. We each insist the other is being selfish. From one corner, he sees our marriage falling apart; from the other, I see him telling me I can't be free.

Our house has become an awkward space, uncomfortable and claustrophobic. I circle around this person who has been waiting for years for me to recover, but now that I'm finally making progress, I want to fly the coop, with or without him. It's unfair.

I want to experience all the things I didn't get to experience before, when I was Lillie's prisoner.

Leon has wanted me to be free from the disorder, so we can live happily in our cozy nest. But I don't want to stay in the nest. I've just discovered I have wings, and I want to fly.

Most couples I know fight about money or jealousy. We fight about my eating disorder and our lacking sex life.

"Can I travel?" I say.

"Sure, you can do whatever you want, but if you go, don't expect me to be here when you get back."

"This is so unfair. You're so needy!" I shut myself in the bathroom, where I look in the closet and see the unopened box of condoms. *Why would I want to have sex with you when I hate you?*

At night, when Leon and I argue, the only places I can go to get away are the bathroom and the kitchen. *Hmm.* The only two places available are the places to begin a binge and end the binge: the refrigerator, the toilet. I feel the walls pressing in around me.

52

TREES ARE MY BALANCE

I'm a tree lover. It's in my blood. Something in me craves their stability, the way they hunker down with their roots in the soil, solid, unmoving. I am like water, carving through rock, constantly changing course. Leon is a tree standing firmly where he's planted. I gravitate towards trees; they are my balance.

Lately I have hope for positive change. With every day that I do not throw up, I feel freer and lighter and closer to the free person I'm striving to become.

As much as I love Leon, as much as he is my balancing tree, the feeling that what I want isn't here has been creeping in. I've been feeling like I need to go somewhere that is dense yet open. Lately I've been dreaming of running through forests of tall redwoods and huge evergreens. Neither of these tree species grows in Hawai'i.

53

PREVENT ME FROM LYING TO MYSELF

"What you're looking for doesn't exist," Leon says. "You could travel the whole, wide world and not find what you're looking for."

But what if it does, and by giving up on it I won't find it?

Love, for me, is synonymous with beauty, happiness, and freedom. When I feel the most free and happy is when I feel the most love. *Feel* the most love, not *know* there is love, but *feel it.*

*

At a personal growth seminar that Leon and I attend as a bonding activity, we partner up for an exercise. The question: "How can I love you?"

My answer: "Let me be free, and show me a different perspective."

Leon's answer: "Constant reassurance."

My husband has always been committed to our marriage, while my energy has been spent trying to survive my eating disorder. It seems that the more I change, the less our old marriage contract is valid. We don't have a new one yet, so we dance around each other frantically, neither one of us getting what we want. My parents are noticing and starting to pry. They ask questions I don't want to answer, because I don't know how. Leon and I try to convince each other that each of our versions of marriage is the right one. It's a no-win situation.

I'm an amalgamation of the new and the old me. Although Leon doesn't want me to have the eating disorder, maybe he does want the old me. Liza warned me that this usually happens. I can't see myself with anyone but Leon, but he also knows all my dirty secrets, and that simple fact makes me want to distance myself from him. I want to start over with someone new who can put distance between the person I am today and the person I used to be.

PART TWO

I can trust myself. I can love myself.
Yes, you can.

54

YES, YOU CAN

I take a trip to visit a friend on the mainland, and I end up meeting a guy. He's unlike most people I've known. When I return to Hawai'i, he becomes a metaphor, an embodiment of all my other choices, my other options, the roads I can't travel because I'm tethered to Leon. My mind wanders to all the possibilities I'm missing. The road not traveled waits with plummy possibility.

"You're so selfish," Leon says. He senses the disconnection—that I'm craving someone who isn't him.

I don't deny that I'm being selfish, because I am. I've come to like the word, because I've never been selfish before. And by selfish, I mean actually doing what I want for myself, not to gain others' approval. I've been the one to sacrifice myself, so others could be content. Now, I refuse to do it anymore.

Religion was black and white. My eating disorder was black and white. Leon is black and white. My parents are black and white. The world seems black and white. I can't live anymore in a world of black and white. I'm afraid it will kill me.

It looks bad. It looks as though I'm interested in pursuing a relationship with another man, because I begin to converse with him. Part of me is, I suppose, even though I know I won't end up with him. It looks very bad. I'm not proud that I let my mind wander and entertain the possibility that my sexual problems can be resolved with someone else. I'm profoundly grateful that he's not in my time zone.

I've tried to keep my conversations with this man secret, but the tension becomes palpable as Leon realizes I'm distracted. I don't know who I am. I feel like a tangled pile of unraveled yarn.

Once a week, Leon and I meet my parents for dinner. Tonight, we're milling around concrete benches outside an Italian restaurant, waiting to be seated, when my dad sits next to me and tells me, "You better smarten up. You're being a selfish bitch, breaking Leon's heart and becoming so new-age-y."

I stand up and walk away. It's my twenty-ninth birthday dinner.

If I'm myself, people won't love me. If I'm true to myself, I'll end up all alone. I walk straight to the bathroom and sit on a closed toilet seat lid to think. When I whisper to myself, "I'm alone," I start to cry.

I do want to be with Leon. I just don't want his marriage boundaries to trap me. I'm happy with Leon, but I'm not happy being confined. If I don't want to leave him, it means I want to stay, but how can I stay if he's going to confine me in a pretty cage.

In spite of everything I'm not doing right, tonight I'm proud of myself. Although my twenty-ninth birthday is spent talking about our crumbling marriage, and although my dad throws shitty comments across the table, when the food is served, I do not binge. I stay present with what is happening, uncomfortable and full, and I do not reach for Lillie to numb me out. *Happy birthday to me.*

*

During therapy, I tell Liza about the incident. She reminds me that when I was a child, fights often happened at the dinner table. I couldn't just get up and leave. "I just want you to notice that," she says, "where the food was, you felt powerless, which might have contributed to you choosing it as your tool to gain power later in life."

*

"I had a Smurf dream last night," my dad says when I walk in their house for our weekly family get-together.

"A Smurf dream?" I say.

"Yeah, one with you riding the Smurf down the hill."

I almost cry. *Hair blowing in the wind, wheels cycling 'round at a frightening speed, the sun streaming through the clouds. Freedom.*

At the dinner table, my dad tells me he's been dreaming of fond memories of when we were close, meaning when I idolized him. He says it like he's mourning the loss of someone who died.

My mom can't get through dinner without bursting into tears. She excuses herself to go to the bathroom. She's crying over my marriage, and I feel like it's my fault. I go and sit outside the bathroom door and talk to her through a small crack. She and my father both blame my friend Di for driving a wedge between Leon and me. I do choose to spend time with Di over spending time with Leon, but it's my choice and my fault, not Di's. The issue of Leon and me not getting along right now has nothing to do with Di. It has to do with me recovering and realizing I have no idea who I am apart from my family, Leon, and Lillie.

Maybe she hears me, but she continues to cry about how much Leon loves me and how much he's sacrificed and put up with. "Leon being hurt is killing me," she says, her voice quivering.

"Oh, OK, so it's my fault?"

"Yes, it's all your fault."

What the hell? I walk away from the door and leave her crying. *How is it my fault when all I'm trying to do is figure out who I am?*

No one's asking me what I want. It's all accusations and "I'm ruining Leon's life." Now that I'm finally establishing boundaries, I've become the source of everyone's pain and sorrow. As long as I remained the same wounded person, everything was OK. But as soon as I start to become someone new in a way that doesn't suit their expectations, suddenly I'm responsible for their unhappiness.

My mom asks, "Do you just want me to step back and give you your own life?"

I have a hard time not exploding. I bare my teeth to keep my tone quiet, but the answer comes out like metal dragging across concrete, "Yes!"

That should have been said a long time ago.

I know my parents love me, so why do they tell me what a bad job I'm doing with my life instead of asking me where I'm coming from? Why don't I get any congratulations for not throwing up seven times a day? I wish they would support me, even if they don't agree with me or understand my compulsion to push away from my marriage.

For the first time in my life, I'm adamantly opposing my family's wishes. I go head-to-head with them. They bring their best weapons, and I don't back down. I refuse to do what they want, even if it means alienating them. For the first time in my whole life, I'm doing something solely for me and listening to my own voice.

Every day I ask myself the same question, "What if I am ruining my life?" I want to be free, but I no longer know what that means or how I get there.

Every day the distance between us increases. Leon pulls me towards him. I push away.

*

Sex is intertwined with eating disorders. I developed anorexia when I was fifteen, and my sexual self is stunted at that age. I've never reached the point my friends talk about, where sex is awesome. I secretly hate my friends a little when they tell me how great sex is. I'm angry at sex. I'm angry at the religion that taught me sex was bad.

Leon, my mom, and my dad try to shove religion in my face as their argument for why I'm a bad person. My dad says I'm lost, and that's why the devil's making his move on me. I'm so sick of fighting with evil that sometimes I don't care. I'm angry at religion for making me feel like I'm never good enough, never enough. If I don't live in religion's little box, then something's wrong with me spiritually. I'm, as my dad says, "running away from God instead of running to Him." *But what if I no longer want to buy into it? What if I believe that God is love?*

I don't like the term New Age, yet I'm starting to use the terminology. Doesn't God love me and accept me? Doesn't He know how much I've suffered on this path and that my intention is not to hurt people? Is it wrong to want autonomy?

When I was little, I knew that I was free, but that was so long ago. I don't remember what it feels like anymore. All I have are fragments, metaphors, hints of memory.

Freedom is a blue Smurf tricycle. Freedom is the wind blowing through my hair, when my arms are outstretched and my face is staring up into the sun on the exhilarating ride downhill. Freedom isn't just holding on for as long as you can.

What should I do?

What do I choose to do?

What do I want to do?

What is the right thing to do?

At work, they're playing Pachelbel's Cannon in D, my wedding song. I sneak into an empty treatment room to cry. I feel sad for the people who love me, because they end up hurt. I'm messed up, and I'm making messes of everything. Eventually, I wander back around the spa and lie to anyone who asks why my eyes look puffy.

My friend Mel, who lives on the mainland, is the most helpful. She doesn't take my side or say anything negative about Leon. She helps me get clarity. "Take away all the religious language and get to what Leon is saying. He's just using Christian terms to express feelings without context. What he might really be saying is, 'I'm feeling left out, hurt, abandoned, or ignored.' Look at what his energy is saying behind his words."

"That's a good point," I say.

"Close your eyes for a second," she says. "Picture yourself in the middle of a football field. The decision to stay with Leon is on one side and the decision not to stay with him is on the other. Which way do you want to go?"

I squint and open my eyes. "I don't know. The problem is that both of them make me almost equally happy. There's a huge part of me that wants to leave and be alone and independent and experience other people. There's a huge pull towards that, towards leaving people. Because, unlike my family, alone, for me, is not a horrible, scary thing. Alone has been a constant my whole life. Sad, yes, but not scary anymore."

"I strongly believe that you've done lifetimes of being alone. Maybe, in this life, you chose Leon so you could work on staying connected and not disconnecting. Think about it. Your growing edge is letting someone in and being seen."

"I know that sexuality and sex factor into this, because the issue is allowing myself to be vulnerable. I associate vulnerable with weak, which equals bad, which equals 'I hate myself for being a pathetic failure.'"

"Whoa, wait. It doesn't have to be sex. I'm talking about letting someone in to see who you are. I feel like the only hope for healthy intimacy is for each person to remain themselves and then have a shared world, too."

"But my instinct is to reject the idea of being one, as a couple, because I was never first my own."

We do our verbal dance. Today, she has the lead and gently twirls me around the room. Before she hangs up, Mel says, "I think you're a complicated, intimately loving individual."

55

THROUGH MY CAGE

Di asks me if I feel unloved, but the weird thing is that whether I'm loved is never my question. I know I'm loved, but I'm also not happy. Since I'm not happy, I must not be getting love in the way I like to receive it.

"You're addicted to new experiences," my friend from college tells me, "and once you're stable, you feel dead,"

"That sounds awful. That means I'm just completely unstable," I say.

He says, "Everything I've loved about you is anti-stability."

"Huh?"

"You're fun. I can be myself around you."

Fun?

"Listen," he says. "It's no secret I was infatuated with you before. But I got over you by thinking about how you changed your life plan, like, every month and how you had fifty thousand things you wanted to do that you were equally passionate about. And about how you didn't want kids. I mean, I'd think about buying us a house, and then you'd say, 'Oh, I decided I wanted to live on a boat for the rest of my life.'"

I laugh into the phone, because I want to cry a little. It's true. My instability has been my only freedom from the cage of my eating disorder. Fun, random adventures were my escape.

"OK, so I just have to say this," he says. "What you're doing to Leon is essentially what my ex-wife did to me. She suddenly realized how she'd had no independence and wanted it all. Basically, she took all the confidence that I gave her, and when she felt OK, she left me."

I've heard him talk about how he loved her, I've heard him call her countless ugly names, and now I'm in the category of selfish, heartless bitch. When he uses the same words for me, they seem unfair, but it doesn't make them less true. When I hang up, I know he's still my friend, and I know he thinks I'm being a bitch and all those other names I won't mention.

*

I'm beginning to want to give up this whole journey of discovering who I am, because all I'm feeling is unhappy and trapped. It terrifies me to know that if I'm not being true to myself, then my eating disorder will get hold of me again. I can't let it happen when I'm just breaking free. I cannot be sucked back in.

Lately, I feel like the woman I'm becoming has been attacked. The only thing that keeps me pushing forward, when it would be easier to surrender, is knowing that if I give in I won't discover who I am. I'll forever be controlled by Lillie, and she won't go away.

56

THE THINGS THAT SCARE ME

Sometimes I wake up at night in the middle of a silent scream. I'm scared that I'm wrong, that everything my family is telling me is true: I'm lost, I'm New Agey, I'm bad, I'm being tricked by Satan. I'm afraid I'm floundering. I'm scared I'm never going to find out who I am. I'm scared of not being allowed to have my own, unique personality. I'm scared everyone's going to leave me. I'm scared I can't do it on my own. I'm scared God's not talking to me. I'm scared I'm going to be punished. I'm scared that if I'm not true to myself, my soul will die. I'm scared if I am myself, I'll no longer have a husband or a relationship with my parents. I'm scared of always being unhappy.

I'm scared to accept myself and love myself. I'm scared of my sadness, my anger, my intensity, and my tendency to self-destruct. I'm scared of consequences. I'm scared of commitment and pretty little cages. I'm scared of doing all this soul-searching and then realizing I'm back where I started. I'm scared of being vulnerable. I'm scared that deep down I'm powerless.

I'm scared of being a failure. I'm afraid I'll spend my whole life just one pathetic leap from the edge of the mountain. I'm scared of sitting alone with myself, because I'm scared I'll get sucked into the black hole of me. I'm scared that the dark will win. I'm afraid my light isn't strong enough. I want to be strong.

57

STRANGE SHAPES

My brother's girlfriend tells me that she likes to think of a relationship as a net. One that can fit all kinds of strange shapes. One that is elastic enough to be able to hold the new, strange shape of each person as the person grows and changes.

Hmm.

*

When I step into Pastor Larry's tiny office, barely big enough to seat three people, my guard is completely up, because I've prepared myself for someone like my father. Pastor Larry is about his age. He's whiter than my dad and has a little less hair, but he's fatherly. As I sit, I start to think maybe it was a bad idea to come here for marriage counseling.

Instead of confirming my distrust, he validates me. He says he hears how sad and confined I feel. "Two independent people choose each other—not out of need or dependence but out of choice." He looks directly into my eyes, "I love you and God loves you. It is for freedom that Christ set us free. God wants to give you the freedom you want. It may come with consequences, if you make bad decisions in your freedom, but God loves you and will always be there for you."

I haven't said a word, because I'm too scared and shocked to open my mouth. If I do, tears will fall out of my eyes likes stones.

He says Leon and I have a common non-negotiable: we believe in God. So we should start there and build. He turns to me again, and says I'm a beautiful woman on the inside and I am loved.

I cry. I can't hold back the tears. Here is an adult telling me God loves me, and He loves me not because I think or feel a certain acceptable way, but because I am me. It's a relief to hear him acknowledge that I'm not crazy to believe it's possible—I can be loved for who I am.

I've experienced this unconditional love with Di. One day, my journal was open on the floor, and while I was sleeping, she covered a blank page with the words, "I love you PERIOD." Unconditional love means to love someone *period*.

Because Pastor Larry is coming from that place of unconditional love, I'm able to hear him when he tells me to seek God and to try to do my best, so I don't make the choices that lead to hurtful consequences. But even if I do make those choices, I am still loved and validated as a person.

*

Choices are all I think about now—about my tendency to self-destruct, about staying with Leon, about the terror of leaving him. I ask myself questions all the time, maybe that's why I'm so exhausted. My mind doesn't know how to shut up.

Until this point, I have never doubted my love or my desire to be with him, so I don't think it's fair to make a decision now. We don't know what will happen. I don't know how much freedom I want or need and if that can work in a marriage. On the other hand, what if I leave and end up feeling just as lonely?

As I look at him, I realize that being married to Leon has allowed me to subdue the voice that says, *You're all alone. No one likes you.*

*

My body reacts as though I'm a vampire fighting the urge for blood. All day long I fight the urge to binge and purge.

I'm fantasizing about the man I met on my trip to the mainland, because something about him reminds me of my first love. All those memories—the ones I kept nicely repressed—are flooding back.

A ridiculous new thought jumps into my head. It tells me that if I have sex with someone else, it might fix the hurt I feel about the past, like homeopathic medicine—like curing like. Another voice keeps circling in my head. *No one will be there for you in the end. You're pushing away the one and only person in your life who wants to commit to you. What a stupid girl.*

Then, stupidly, I keep going down the spiral.

58

THE PROBLEM WITH ME

Numbing out comes easily to me. *Poof.* I can go to a little space in my head where my heart is cold and I cannot feel.

"Are you still in love with me?" Leon asks.

"Love, to me, is freedom and happiness, and I'm not feeling those right now, so . . ."

"So you don't love me?"

My view is murky. I know I love him, but it's like the kind of love I know I have for my parents. I know I love him, so why can't I feel anything to back that up? "I feel claustrophobic. Sometimes I feel like, in order to know myself, I need to be alone to figure out who I am."

The silence sometimes is worse than words, because there is so much anxiety that fills it.

My mind churns: *I'm a bad person. I hurt people. I lie. I harbor an ocean of guilt. I've deceived people. I haven't been real. My smile is a costume. I lie. I love myself. I lie. I want to love myself. But I'm a bad person.*

Leon's text reads: "If you truly loved me, you wouldn't be hurting me."

The numbness turns to feeling that pours into my heart and belly. Guilt drowns me. *Why am I doing this to him? It hurts. It hurts. It hurts.* Part of me is letting go, and the other part of me is trying to find a way to hold on that will allow me to feel free. *Either choice makes me feel like I'm dying inside.*

From: Leon
To: Christen
I feel like it needs to be said:

It's OK that you have an eating disorder. It's OK, even though part of you felt trapped your whole life, never having the chance to discover yourself because you had a mask for every circumstance. It's OK. It's OK that people, although lost, made your life hard by making fun of you, by not taking you seriously, by not approving of what you do or who you are. It's OK. It's OK that you're "flawed." It's OK. It's OK to be angry. It's OK to be sad. It's OK to be lonely. It's OK to struggle. It's OK, Christen. God loves you unconditionally. I love you unconditionally— so much so that I would let you go if that's what you wanted.

I just want you to know that it's OK. It's not easy, but it's OK.

Eternally,
Leon

It's a real problem that I sabotage myself. A voice inside tells me, *You're worthless. You don't deserve to be happy. You deserve to suffer.*

59

WHAT I DID TODAY FOR PLEASURE

"If space or freedom is so important to you, go find it. Don't stay in the house and treat me like shit because I'm invading your space."

I wake up to see these words written on the mirror.

Leon stands in the doorway and tells me how lucky I am to be with him, how I have it made. He complains that I haven't been making his meals or cleaning the house. "I'm in the kitchen all night studying for us," he says.

How unfair. I don't appreciate this. I went to work all day for us.

"I want a wife," he says. "Someone who's going to be there for me. Someone who wants to be there and choose me. Not someone who's going to live this double life."

I want to choose Leon, but I also want to be a nomad. Maybe I was never meant to be married.

The guy I met on vacation tells me that if I can channel my energy away from guilt and into pleasure, it will be powerful. "What we give to others is what we usually want to receive, so we have to be able to give it to ourselves. If we can't first maintain the space for ourselves, then no one is going to be able to meet us there." He says I can start by taking some time every day to do one thing for the sake of pleasure.

Just that word, *pleasure,* conjures an unpleasant, guilty, sexual sensation in me. My mind goes *bad, dirty, wrong* before I can stop it.

When I go to work at the spa, I want to die. I feel the same exhaustion, numbness, and depression I used to feel in high school, when I wrote wistful poems about the free fall from an ocean cliff to the jagged rocks below. *Why does the fucking phone keep ringing?* I want to cry but I can't.

I'm informed that if I'm not in uniform, my appointments will be shifted to other staff members. "Maybe that will get your attention," I'm told. I glance down at my faded yellow slippers. My chest swells with anger like a rubber band expanding and releasing with a snap.

I'd like to punch someone in the face. Fuck my fucking shoes. They're fucking shoes. My life is falling apart, and I'm being scolded about my shoes? I should take three steps and smash the stupid ringing phone into her face, wrap the chord around her neck, choke her until she hits the floor unconscious, and walk away peacefully as my flip-flops slip-slap the floor on the way out. Instead, I nod politely and plop a raspberry in my mouth.

My whole life, I've followed the path others chose for me. *Just tell me that I'm good and that you approve of me, and all the pain will be worth it. Then it will be worth everything I ignore in myself.*

I smile to myself as I cross one leg over the other, my little yellow slipper hanging from my foot. I take pleasure in every little *Fuck you* I get to deliver in hidden ways. I'm not going to live up to the potential people see in me. I'm going to be a little difficult, or a lot, because I'm smart and articulate and I can play life's stupid, boring game with a perfect pretend smile, because people don't know me at all. And somehow I know this scares them.

And that's what I did today for pleasure.

*

I force my mind to stop churning when I have clients. I shut out all the pain in my body so that it doesn't transfer to them, because I cannot, will not, give my clients any of this. Even today, when I'm not in the mood to be serving clients, I pull it together. "Hi," I say, "my name is Z. I'll be doing your service today." I smile even though I feel like crying.

When I come back into the treatment room I think, *OK. Fifty minutes. I can do this.* The lights are dim as I turn my steamer on for her facial and place my hands on her temples.

"Can you focus on my neck and under my chin," she says.

"Yes, I can do that," I answer softly, criticizing myself for judging her for being another superficial person.

"My husband's funeral is tomorrow, and everything's starting to sag," she says.

My heart shudders like a bullet has passed through it, and suddenly I'm not in my head at all. I'm right here in this moment with her. I cup my hands over her eyes and hold back the tremor in my voice. "I'm so sorry," I say.

"Thank you," she says.

My only thought, as I hold my hands over her, is to transfer love. *Love love love love.* For the next fifty minutes, the goal of my life, my only goal, is to love her and to be completely focused on her. We don't speak at all for the entire time.

When she exits the room and I'm there holding a glass of water for her, she says, "Thank you. That felt wonderful. I've been so stressed out lately."

I hug her, because I don't know what to say. "I'll be thinking of you tomorrow," I tell her.

As I watch her walk down the shadowy hallway, the thoughts resume. *You are such a bad person.* Part of me believes it, because I think I should be able to know what's going on with people. She'd come in smiling and cheerful, and I'd had no idea.

"You should feel guilty," Lillie says. "You're bad and selfish."

"Shut up," I say out loud, and then look around in a small panic to see if anyone heard me.

60

COLLIDE

As I drive home, the sun is an orange ball sinking under the clouds behind rays of light. With the cold wind in my face, windows down, I sing to Ani Difranco, wishing for miles of open road and enough gas to keep me going for hours. When I pick up Leon, I can tell he's feeling resentful, because he gives only one-word answers to my questions. When we get to my parents' house for dinner, I park, and he immediately heads inside without waiting for me.

My parents' house, the house I grew up in, is cozy. The small Christmas tree on the kitchen counter is lit with colored lights. Food's cooking. Music's playing. We have a delicious dinner, and afterwards my parents want us to open our presents early. They give us stockings filled with a book, a picture frame, a candle, and some money with a note telling us to spend it together.

Later, my father walks by and spies me in the bathroom picking my face, which I've done since I was a little kid. He gives me the stink eye.

"What?" I say. "Why are you looking at me like that? It's my face. I can do whatever I want with it."

He furrows his brow. "Why are you so angry. You're so hateful. You never used to be like this. I feel like I lost four people this year." He names three people who have died, ". . . and you."

My mind floods with multiple responses that leave me exhausted and speechless. I shut down and stand there not saying anything. *How do I explain that I'm realizing I never liked myself much before, and I don't want to be that person again?*

Since the house is small, everyone hears our conversation, and my mom jumps in and starts talking about nice, happy things, trying to pretend everything is nice. It makes me even sadder.

Before we leave, I peek into the dark computer room where my dad sits on a small chair with his face lit up by the screen. He doesn't look at me, but I can tell his eyes are teary, and it breaks my heart that I don't know how to begin to talk to him. Everyone is suffering.

As Leon drives home, I stare out the window at the moon in the dark sky. I just want everyone to leave me the hell alone. I want my mom and my dad and Leon to leave me in peace.

*

One of my friends says I'm shaking the foundations of who everyone thinks I am.

"But what if I want to change who I am?"

"No one likes change," he says and then laughs, "except for you, because you like to change all the time."

Hmm. If that's how I'm perceived, then perhaps I should work on appearing—no, *being*— more stable. Maybe I should work on staying with Leon, because my tendency—no, my *compulsion*—is to run, escape, reinvent myself when anyone gets too close.

My brother tells me that I have to show and tell Leon the new plan I want for my life and see if he wants to go along with me, now that my plan has changed.

"Do you even want him to accompany you anymore in life?" My brother tells me he asked his girlfriend the other day, "Do you like my land?" and she responded, "I like where you are."

Leon and I once had that kind of love, and I am responsible for pushing it away. We don't talk much, now, because it ends in fights and frustrations. He knows what he wants, and I can't decide.

The therapy-like marriage counseling that we've been going to is giving me less hope that we'll stay together, because of how much I want to focus on myself and how far apart we've grown around every fundamental belief system, starting with religion.

*

A friend's bridal shower is held at a fancy hotel with tea and mini sandwiches. I hand her gifts to open, so I can push down the uncomfortable feeling that I don't belong. I realize I am unlike other women.

I told my husband if he bought me a wedding ring, I wouldn't marry him.

My friend opens up a china set and everyone ohhs and ahhs. I find myself thinking, *I wouldn't want a china set. A china set implies that you have a special cabinet to put it in and a family to hand it down to. That's the last thing I want. I'm anti-stability, remember?*

*

That night, at our weekly family dinner, my dad and I have an after-dinner conversation in the driveway. It's a masculine arguing match. I'm swearing, and he's dissing my friends, and we get teary-eyed about our past anxiety attacks and my eating disorder and how I feel like God didn't answer my prayers. "You're fighting a spiritual battle," he says.

"I'm not denying it, but what I am fighting for is to get to the middle, which is where I want to be. I need a balance." I try to explain myself.

He proceeds to tell me how I feel. "Because you're dark, you want to live in the darkness."

"I don't want to live in darkness."

"You only hear what you want to," he says. "Look at what you're doing. You're selfish."

"Whatever. This is where I'm insulted and leaving," I say and walk away.

"Oh, how New Agey. Yeah, walk away. You're good at that."

*

Later that evening, when Leon and I are in our kitchen making popcorn, my dad calls me with tears in his voice. "I want you to know that I love you so much. Do you know that?"

"Yes. I know," I say. I can't deny it, because I know it's true, but sometimes I wonder how I'm supposed to survive the love of the people who love me. Of course I feel guilty. When my dad cries, my heart cracks. It's like watching someone kick a puppy.

As I hang up and plunk down on the couch, Leon makes it worse by telling me, "Guilt is there for a reason, because it's God's conscience in us."

That's my favorite one, because I've felt guilty for everything my whole life. I am *not* feeling guilty anymore. My hand angrily shoves popcorn into my mouth as Leon flicks on the TV. *You didn't have a hard life. You don't deserve to be messed up.*

Leon clicks angrily through the channels. "You act like you've had a hard life," he says. When I pick up my pen to write down his words, he finishes with, "What? Are you going to write that down to tell your therapist?" He throws the remote down on the bed and walks into the bathroom, separating us with the door.

In my journal I write: "FUCK YOU! FUCK YOU! FUCK YOU! YOU DON'T FUCKING KNOW ME! FUCK YOU!"

Then I watch *Food, Inc.*, and that makes me even more disheartened about humanity. If we treat animals that horribly, is there any hope for the way we treat each other?

61

IF IT'S NOT A YES

"If it's not a yes, it's a no. Stop dragging your feet." My client at work tells me this is exactly what her mom told her when she was eighteen and deciding whether she wanted to get married. She decided yes.

For Christmas, Leon and I take a vacation and go and visit his dad and his grandmother. They live where it's cold and snowy. My husband spent his childhood growing up in this weather, but I've seen snow only once, because I was born and raised in Hawai'i. In the past, his family has not seen the best of me. I'm a loving person, but it's incredibly difficult to pretend like I don't have an eating disorder and be on my best behavior. The eating disorder made me edgy, moody, and unpredictable to be around. I'm determined to change, and yet on this trip, our marriage hangs in the balance. Why? I know the answer. Me. I could make a ton of excuses in my defense, but they would be candy-coated lies.

I know I'm doing this to myself. Leon wants to be in this marriage, and I am all over the place. I'm not going to lie; I have a dangerous fascination with the guy I met on vacation, and I'm still communicating with him. Because we are so different, I think we can learn something from each other. One part of me confuses his personality traits with a man I once loved. Another part of me is aware of my tendency to swagger towards my demise while convincing myself I'm doing what's good for me.

The tension around us is tactile—taking form as though a dark shadow is present in the room, a shadow on the verge of releasing all my secrets into the silence. Leon and I fight. A lot. He asks me angrily, "What are you waiting for? Just make your decision, already, instead of keeping me holding on." He tells me that he sees the road I'm crossing, and I have only one foot on our side. He says I'm going to find out that the people I think are my friends are not what they appear to be.

My stomach drops, the same way it does when my father talks to me and I feel the anxiety, conflict, and self-doubt. All I want is myself.

I can tell that Leon's twenty-one-year-old sister is crying in the bathroom. Everyone in the house knows. Our marital problems are no secret. When his sister emerges from the bathroom she hugs me and tells me, "We love you, too." When she walks away I burst into tears. She can see how much her brother is hurting because of me, and yet told me she loves me, too.

I don't get it. Leon's family can see that I'm hurting him, yet they still act lovingly towards me.

His grandmother comes and sits on the couch across from me. "The travels in your eyes . . ." she says. "I want a video camera drilled into your head. It looks like I should be able to look into your eyes and hear and see everything. You can tell a lot by looking into someone's eyes and yours . . . are busy." She smiles warmly.

I know what she is seeing. She's seeing how my brain diverts to fifty things at once, how I have many conversations going on simultaneously, and how I don't know how to make them stop so I can have a second of peace. *How can she see that? Why are they being nice to me?* Outside it's snowing. Soft little snowflakes pour down from the sky.

"Do you want to take off your coat?"

"No," I shrug. "I'm cold," I tell Leon's grandmother, touching the windowpane with my fingertips, knowing I'll probably wear my coat the whole time I'm here, whether I'm indoors or out.

Outside, the ground is white, soft, and peacefully silent. The branches of the skeleton trees are dusted with white snowflakes hovering on their branches. Maybe my life is becoming more like this, a cold fresh exhale, a cloud of visible air, clearing out to make way for the pleasant silence. It's the stillness where God waits patiently for us to enter, to let the breath flow in and out of us, clearing away our sins, making our insides white as snow. I need to start praying again.

62

CHOICES

Leon has been spying on me, going through the phone records. He tells me he's keeping tabs on me. "I know you've been texting him and lying about it," he says.

"Yeah," I say, "because when I did tell you, that one night, you flipped out on me."

"If this continues, then I'm canceling your texting plan and you can get your own phone."

Sure. That makes me want to be honest. Aggression and force are both ways to my heart. Not.

"Can I go back to visit?" I say looking up from my book.

"You can, but my answer stands. If you go, we're getting a divorce," he says.

"What if I just went to see my friend?"

"Stop lying to yourself," he says from the opposite couch. "You're not going to go there and just see your friend. The reason you want to go is to see that guy."

I do want to see my friend, but Leon may be right. Even if I have no intention of seeing the guy I met on vacation, if he were nearby, I think I'd end up seeing him as well. I can't figure out why this is so important. It's as if I'm staking my marriage on this decision for no real reason other than the principle of getting my way.

"I don't want to talk about this anymore. You know my answer." he says and goes back to reading his book.

When we return to Hawai'i, I'm going to resent him for this. I'm going to pull away even more. Why am I staying? Because he takes care of me? Because I'm afraid to be alone? Because we do have fun together? Because we have history? Because we were once so in love?

My brother once told me, "These people know you through huge vital points in your life, and they share those memories. If you're no longer with them, no one knows who you are."

Leon looks up. "I'm reading books on marriage, and you are reading books on auras," he says, as if that explains everything.

*

Last night, I couldn't sleep. I lay in bed for three hours staring at the ceiling. There are so many other paths. The pull is appealing. Although I don't know what I expect to find, I can't fully commit to Leon unless I solve this dilemma.

His stance is that I absolutely cannot go back to the place where I met the man who so intrigues me, where alternate paths lie. Leon says this is the last straw, this is his line in the sand. He's come across half of the beach, and this is his line. Then the anger and frustration get the better of him, and he rants, "Why am I fighting at all anymore?"

I feel like I'm drowning. Even if I choose him, I'm still going to feel constricted, because my path seems so different from his. I'm scared of struggling alone, and I do want to know that someone's there to take care of me. I want to be happy.

Because it's cold, because we're indoors, these conversations happen around food. We're arguing and eating popcorn, and Lillie snaps, "Screw this. Binge and purge." The conversations nauseate me, and when I eat too much, my stomach hurts like it's being pierced.

I am hurting him. Leon doesn't have what I want or need. At this point, I can't give him what he wants. Silence is an answer. If I cannot voice the word *yes,* then by default my answer is *no.*

63

MY HAPPY NEW YEAR

I hardly ever cry . . . and I can't stop crying. I realize how much I feel trapped by making the decision not to go. I feel like I'm dying inside, like my soul is telling me I made the wrong decision to stay with Leon. I'm nauseated. My head hurts. There's so much pressure. I want to throw up. My body is seized by tremors. I can't stop crying. I never cry. I never cry in front of other people. I want to go. I want to be free and whole.

I down two shots of tequila. My body feels heavy. I can't stop crying. Alcohol doesn't numb the pain. My body is radiating heat. My neck hurts. A deep soul sadness won't be contained. It overflows. I want peace and happiness. I want the voice in my head to stop screaming.

My friend Mel's advice keeps running through my head, "Go through the hate to get to the love. Go through the hate to get to the love."

The nausea kicks in, and my whole body regurgitates itself. I throw up and come back downstairs to shoot more clear tequila, because I can't stop shaking. Tequila sucks, because it doesn't numb me. Food is my drug of choice, but I'm not in control, because I'm in someone else's house.

My dad calls. Why I pick up is a mystery to me, but I do, like a trained rat. He wishes me a happy new year.

I'd like to put on my fake self, but it's too much effort. My voice that answers is a monotone.

"Are you OK?" he asks.

There's a long pause while I fight to make my voice normal, without the quiver of crying, without weakness. It goes around, this same game we play with his love and his judgment. It ends with both of us on opposite sides arguing almost the same point while treating each other like the enemy.

I find myself pleading with him to let me get off the phone, as if he's holding me hostage. "I don't want to talk anymore, please."

"Why are you being like this?" he says. "What happened to you? We used to be such good friends."

Please, let me get off the phone. I know you love me. Stop, please.

"Are you willing to risk your marriage for yourself?" he asks. It sounds like a trick question.

I've made my choice, even though I'm trying to keep one and find the other. "Yes," I reply. *I'm willing to risk everything. Isn't that clear?*

"You don't even love yourself," he answers, as if calling me out on a lie.

Of course I love myself. Otherwise, why would I be pushing so hard against the three people closest to me, risking all my safety nets, my family, my marriage? Risking it all to find me. My fear is: who I become if I'm not loving myself and being true to myself.

At last, I get off the phone. I find myself on the living room carpet on my hands and knees like a werewolf about to turn. I'm crying to the point of hyperventilating, gasping for air, whispering to myself, "You have to breathe. Slow down. Breathe. Just relax. Calm down. Calm down."

I hug the floor, my face pressing into rough fibers smelling of people's shoes. I wish I were dead. It would be so much easier not to have to deal with this, but then I'd be the loser who accomplished nothing with my life and simply opted out. *Damn it.*

My frantic lungs stop gasping. I wipe my face with the sleeve of my yellow jacket, the color of happiness.

Downstairs, Leon's sister turns to look at me. I avert my eyes, go straight for the countertop and the shot glass and the bottle, shoot, chase, and pour immediately again. My husband's dad gives me a look as he takes a shot and asks if I'm OK. Since I can't talk without crying, I shake my head no. Leon is standing behind me. I can feel his energy pushing against my back. His dad flicks his head, his chin pointing over my shoulder, "You can take the hug he's offering." Again I shake my head no and pour another. *Don't touch me. I hate you right now. I hate how much you love me even though I'm hurting you in completely unfair ways. You still have no idea what I'm going through.*

Watching another movie is beyond awkward as I keep waiting for someone to make me talk, but in this family they do not, and I'm not used to that. Sitting on the couch, I look like a polar bear. I'm shaking as if my clothes were made of ice, and I can't stop the silent tears from sliding down my cheeks. There are no more words. *What is tequila good for, if it doesn't make you numb? Happy New Year.*

*

After the movie, I slink into the shower where the water is either scalding hot or cold. Right now it's scalding hot, so hot I can't stand it. I have to sit down and curl up like a fairy on a mushroom with hot rain pouring down over me. This is what I used to do when I was depressed: take long showers in the dark and pretend I was sitting on the sidewalk and it was raining and my scene was about to start.

The mirrors are completely fogged, so I can't see myself as I brush my teeth.

In my room, on my pillow, there's a note from Leon. "I love you, despite what you think, more than dirt"—an old inside joke meaning that he loves me more than the sustenance of all things. With no emotion I remove it from my pillowcase and toss it on the desk. *My heart is full of so much hate, and I don't want my heart to be full of hate.*

My friend Mel's voice rings in my ears again, "Sometimes you have to go through the hate to get to the love."

So, I sit on my bed and write, because I love words, because they hold so much pain and redemption, because they let me bleed all my spirit into a black stain on a fresh white page. And in that catharsis, I am liberated, separated from myself. I'm merely the playwright of this scene. *Sometimes you have to go through the hate to get to the love.*

And so I write. Until the moment it all has emptied out, and there is silence, and I reach somewhere where I can touch the love—even if it barely grazes my fingertips.

64

SEPARATENESS

I continue communicating with the guy from vacation, continue being detached, continue wanting to travel, and Leon reaches his breaking point.

"I can't do this anymore," he says. "I'll make it as easy as I can for you to move out. You can have the savings. You can have the car."

I'm crying, crying, crying. We're not going to be together. This is what part of me wants, and yet it feels like I'm losing. The other part of me is wild, frantic, scared, hopeless, and torn. *If I want my freedom, then why doesn't all of me want it? Who's going to watch* The Simpsons *with me? Who's going to eat popcorn and laugh and be cute with me as if we were little kids? Maybe I can change. Yes, I can change. No, I can't change. I don't know.*

He says he can't go through another semester, with me on the phone talking to other people, while his grades suffer. He can't concentrate on his own life. What he says is fair.

It's fair, but that doesn't stop me from crying. I've been following my own road, yet the reality at the end comes as a shock. *Oh, my God.* I'm sobbing violently with a ball of tissue next to my leg.

Leon says, "All I want is that snapshot of us in Tahiti." It's a picture of the future. We are old, and we're walking along the beach, holding hands and smiling at each other, in our own world.

Guilt rips through my heart, because when I try to see the picture, he's not there. We're not the way we used to be—happy together.

When I apologize, he shrugs, "I'm kinda numb. I've done a lot of crying about it already. The truth is I feel like I've already lost you."

My huge coat makes me feel like a blue marshmallow as I step into the cold silence of the street. In the dark, the streetlights filter down an orange glow while my boots crunch into the snow-covered pavement like the sound of biting into an apple. Outside, I am the only thing moving. Nothing lives out here, no birds, no sound. It's like being in a life-sized snow globe.

I've read that freezing to death isn't horrible, that you get numb and tired and go to sleep. I think about taking off all my clothes and burying myself in the yard. *How long would it take me to die?* Because I'm from Hawai'i, probably less that half the time it would take a Midwesterner; too bad I hate the cold. I keep walking past the houses on the block as the air slithers past my neck and into my pockets where I stuff my hands. Small conglomerations of Christmas decorations, like tiny, disjointed families, are displayed on a few snowy lawns. Colored lights flicker against the white backdrop, igniting for a few seconds at a time. The lights blur into rainbow halos through my tears. I wonder if they'll freeze in tiny crystals on each eyelash.

At the end of the block, I'm too cold to continue on. I don't want to get lost wandering the neighborhood.

What are the implications of us not being together? The perfect little girl in me says, *You should call your parents and let them know.* I take a right by the park and fiddle with my phone, but the buttons are difficult to push because my hands are so cold. My feet stamp the snow in place as I settle on a spot next to a tree with bark that makes me want to scrape it with my fingernails. There is silence, then ringing, and my dad picks up.

"Leon and I just separated," I say.

During a long pause, I can feel his disapproval seeping through the phone.

"I think you're making the wrong decision. Leon loves you. The list of pros and cons has many more pros than cons."

The words that follow dissipate as soon as I hear them. My frozen fingers hold the phone as I look at my boots in the snow—my brown boots with the colorful beaded flowers etched into them—and the tree, strong and sturdy and unmoving, in front of me.

When I hang up, I hug the tree. If God were looking, he'd see a little blue marshmallow with little brown boots pressed against the bark of a skeleton tree, and He might wonder who is holding whom.

Sobbing, I pace back down the block kicking piles of snow. *No one understands me.*

No one understands what having an eating disorder for eleven years does to a person. No one understands how much I'll risk for freedom, even if I destroy everything around me. I don't want to, but I don't know how not to. What if I'm being self-destructive solely because it's my pattern? Already I'm wondering if I'll get a second chance.

I stamp my boots into the house, after wiping the evidence of my pain from my face. Leon's dad stands peacefully in the doorway. "Do you know what you're trying to become, what you are searching for, or are you just blindly going out in the dark?"

My hands hurt as they start to defrost, and a tingly feeling sweeps through them, the discomfort of reviving. My fist opens and closes. My long fingers spread out, retract. "In the dark," I say. "I'm blindly going out in the dark."

65

JUST BE

Back in Hawai'i, my mom and dad and Leon and I wait outside CPK with our little buzzer. Leon and I are a few steps from the entrance, and my parents, when he asks me about the conversations that he went searching for and found on my computer. He asks me point-blank: did the conversations concern sex.

I say, "Yes and no."

"It's over," he says. "I can't do this anymore. We're separated."

We've been going back and forth about this for exactly two weeks since my walk in the snow, but I know in an instant that this time he's serious. I can hear it in his voice and see it in the disgust on his face. He has already separated himself from me.

He walks away just as the buzzer lights up in my hand. I feel dirty holding it, like a prize that I want to give back. A smiling girl dressed in black ushers us down the aisle of the crowded restaurant as if in a dream sequence.

At the table, over dinner, my dad calls us both idiots and stares daggers at the side of my head, while my mom pains herself to make polite conversation. Leon looks exhausted, and I can't focus on anything except the stupid voices in my head that won't shut up and the nausea that overtakes me. I swallow my sandwich wishing I could taste it. I haven't been eating much since we returned, maybe an apple and a veggie sandwich a day. A couple of times I wanted to binge and throw up.

My father looks away from me for the rest of dinner, ignoring me as though I'm not even there, except when he shoves me that look that says he's completely disappointed in me.

On the ride home, my mind reviews my dad's silent stare. His look of disgust is burned into my memory.

"What's your plan?" Leon asks breaking the silence.

Plan?

"Can you be out of the house in two weeks or as soon as possible?" he says, adding, "If it was up to me you'd be out tonight."

Wait. What? Who is it up to? Two weeks! Holy shit.

In crisis situations, I go numb. My emotions linger outside the feeling zone, as though I push them away for self-preservation.

Two weeks. Oh, my God, this is happening.

"Isn't this what you wanted?" Lillie asks.

Yes, but I didn't want it this way.

"What the hell do you want then?"

I want to be happy and free.

"Well, now you're free. The happy part is up to you."

But what if I find it's not what I want?

"You should have thought of that before you started," Lillie sings.

Shut up.

*

I begin to look for places to live. I begin to pack my things while Leon's out. I sob because I feel like God's just watching me and doing nothing. *Why won't You talk to me? Please tell me what to do, and I'll do it.* I'm terrified of making the wrong decision, blowing it all, and having God be disappointed in me.

Leon's being firm about wanting me out of the house. I need time to figure myself out, but if we separate and I want to come back as soon as next week, Leon doesn't know if he can take me back.

This whole black-and-white way of thinking makes me crazy. I'm losing my husband and my best friend. He's so cold and forceful. I almost have a breakdown in the kitchen when he explains that I'll be getting my own phone and car insurance for the car. This is not feeling like a separation; this is feeling like a divorce. The woman who wants to travel the world is afraid to move out and pay her own bills and find her own place. I'm the same girl I was in high school. Ten years later, I'm the same girl who is terrified of the world.

"By the way," Leon says, "your dad says he wants your box out of their house."

My brother and I each have a huge plastic box that we store at our parents' house. Mine contains drawing and writings from my childhood.

Leon pauses. "He said it out of anger, though. He probably didn't mean it."

Our home is a small studio, so the kitchen and the bathroom have once again become the only private places where I can escape. Tonight the kitchen wins, because when I hear about my storage box, I can't make it the extra few steps to the bathroom before I start crying. I don't want Leon to see me cry.

Why does my dad have to be so mean when I don't do what he thinks is best? It's as though he were saying, *Could you please remove your box of childhood things from my space? I don't want to see them and be reminded of what a disappointment you are to me.* It feels like my dad is breaking up with me, too, when all that reminds him of me is packed into a box and left outside for me to pick up. Inevitably, the one holding the box feels like she's been thrown out in the trash.

66

THE CHALLENGE OF WARRIORSHIP

Since I'm not welcome in my home with Leon, I go to my parents' house, where I am quasi-welcome. Mentally, it's like a rough train ride through many busy cities with lots of stops and people getting on and off and children shrieking and hundreds of footsteps and coins clanking and coats rustling and the scrape of metal on metal. It's hard to sleep.

I get up and make a piece of toast with ginger and butter. My mom comes into the kitchen and massages my head and face, which gives her an excuse to ask me questions and tell me she doesn't understand what's going on with me.

Hell if I can explain it.

My cat, Comet, who lives at my parents' house, sits at the foot of my bed staring out the window into the darkness of the night. *What is it that she's looking at? Why does she stare at it so intently?* I fall asleep.

When I wake, Comet's sitting on my chest staring at me as if I have the answer to some mysterious question.

I pack some apples and head out, as my mom asks, "You're not still talking to that guy from the vacation, are you?"

My dad mutters something about how I shouldn't be texting at all.

The sky is orange and speckled with poufy cotton-ball clouds. It's still early and peaceful. I'm thankful that I can hold two emotions at once. I can feel horribly sad *and* excited. I love Leon *and* I also love myself. I can separate my two worlds, so I can fully exist in one at the same time I exist in the other.

*

Di and I have spent the past two nights at her parents' house. Lounging in her room reminds me of slumber parties when I was a kid. For a while I lose myself completely in the laughter and innocence, until we must set our alarms for work, and I remember I no longer get to be young and free of responsibilities.

After we both get off work, Di sets up her massage table in her backyard and gives me a massage under the palm trees after sunset as the wind whips across the bay. I wrap up in purple sheets and head to the outdoor shower that overlooks the water. I make us sandwiches with good bread and avocado and think about tomorrow when I'll pack my belongings to leave Leon.

I overhear as Di's mom takes her aside and tells her that I'm welcome to stay as long as I like. My heart melts. *They're going to let me stay? No questions asked? Wow.*

There is no way to be prepared to move out of a house, away from the person with whom I've shared the last six years of my life. There are logistics, like: *Where am I going to put all my things? What the hell am I doing with my life?* I look around the silent house and realize I don't want to leave, but I must. I'm already doing it.

It's not about what to take and what to divide. It's the realization that, with each item I move out of our house, my life as I know it is ending. It's possible that Leon will move on. *What did I set in motion? Did I think this through? Or am I just like my cat, sitting near the window, staring blankly, eyes fixated on a point in the darkness?*

I pull myself together and drive to my parents' house. For some reason they pick tonight to be exceptionally pushy and guilt-provoking. Because the house is so small and there is nowhere to get away from them, I do the only thing I can think of, the only thing I have never tried before. I leave.

And the weird thing? I can see that they expect me to stay there and take it, like a good girl.

I don't know where to go, because I've never left before. It's late, almost eleven o'clock in the evening, so I drive to the closest, safest place I can think of—the street where Leon and I lived. I crawl into the back seat of the car under the bright streetlight and cry while I listen to music and shiver in the cold.

I contemplate going to what used to be our house. I think about what I would say. *Yes, I do want to be together, but I just don't see that working out right now.* What if I tell him I have nowhere to go and ask if can I sleep there? What if he says, *Too bad, but this is your fault,* and shuts the door in my face?

No one likes rejection. I despise it. Tonight, when I'm barely holding on, I don't think I can handle it if the door shuts in my face. I can't handle any snide or mean or guilt-dripping comments, so I stay in my cold car, even as my leg muscles cramp. I realize I would negotiate things I'd never dreamed of for a warm blanket.

When morning comes, the car battery is dead, because I accidentally left the lights on all night. The walk up the driveway is like the walk of shame, as is knocking on Leon's door at seven o'clock and asking him for a jump-start.

67

MY NEW HOUSE

The past week I have been living at Di's house and looking for apartments. Tonight, I'm floundering when I receive a phone call saying my application to rent the house that I thought was a sure thing was rejected. "What am I going to do? I have to have my things out of Leon's house in two days."

Di shoves me her computer. "Don't worry. It'll be fine. Look on Craigslist. I'm going to take a shower."

When she walks back in the room I spin the computer around. "I know this person," I say. "I met him a couple months ago, and we had an awesome conversation."

At ten o'clock the next morning, Di's phone beeps loudly, and we roll over grumpily. "Holy crap, friend, wake up," she says anxiously, jutting up, fully awake. "He absolutely remembers you and thinks you would be a great addition to his house and wants to know if you can come and look at it today."

Thirty minutes later, Di and I are hugging my new landlord in the driveway. The room has a king-size bed. I've always wanted to have one all to myself. I admire the huge windows and dark brown walls. It's peaceful here, like a bear cave, with good energy. Di nods her head. Thirty minutes after that, I'm signing a lease.

Alone in my new room, I glance around at all my things in piles. I didn't have boxes, so the two friends who helped me move threw all my things in our two cars, and we carried them up in a hundred little trips. My mood is melancholy. The reality of moving has set in, because it's final; I just signed a rent check. The reality of our separate lives sinks in. I love Leon. I *love* him, and I'm scared. By doing this, I've ensured that we won't be together, that even if I figure myself out, he won't take me back. The reality overtakes me as I unpack. At our house, everything had its place, but not here. Here, nothing has a home, and it's odd having all my things scattered in piles.

When I brush my teeth at night, I stare into the mirror with a blank expression. When I was little, I was fascinated with the triple mirror in my parents' bathroom. I could tilt the segments inwards, and my reflection would go on forever—a kaleidoscope of me, shifting as I moved. Here, there's only one mirror, large and flat and showing me as I am, searching.

Even though my room is disorganized, the first thing I do is set up the bookshelves along the picture window, so I can light a bunch of candles and watch them burn down as I fall asleep. With the lights off, the flames dance, the shadows of their slender necks and sensual curves slithering on the ceiling. A surge of happiness sweeps through me. My first apartment of my own, my own big bed, my own closet. Everything is completely mine.

"Thank you, Jesus," I whisper out loud, because I can. "Please protect this whole room and fill it with love and peace and positive energy. Thank you for taking care of me. I feel loved by you. Thank you. Thank you. Amen."

I sleep in the middle of my huge bed, equidistant from both sides. My water glass sits on one side table, my music and my journal on the other. The window spans half of the wall space on the right side of my bed and my door opens to the hallway on the other side. I'm proud of myself. When I write in my journal, I recognize that not so long ago I thought I'd never be free of the binging and purging, or the fear of never having enough, of being empty and then overfull and making myself empty again only to want more. Now, I can stay present and experience strong emotions and ride the wave, instead of absorbing them and then throwing them up to make them go away.

In the lower left corner of the mirror that hangs above my headboard, I tape a photo of Leon and me, when we were happy. I sit in the middle of my bed and feel empty and feel what empty feels like and cry and feel hopeless and alone. I also allow myself to feel grateful, to feel the rush of bliss that overtakes me. I know that I am loved by God and He makes all things beautiful in His time.

68

THE PRAYERS WE SAY

Conversations with my father are like fighting over a ball of yarn, with one of us trying to unwind it and the other trying to tie it nicely back up. It gets tangled and knotted until we both end up throwing it to the floor and walking away.

I spend two hours confused and irritated about car and medical insurance and asking why he thinks it's wrong for me to study with a shaman.

My father tells me that I'm going away from God.

*

I stop by Leon's house to get a blanket, and I can barely stop crying to make it out the door. He calls me on my way home and talks to me, which only confuses me and lights a fire to all the rubbish already blowing around in my head. I crumple in my car, my shirt wet and dirty from wiping my nose.

My feet shuffle zombie-like as I extract the huge pillowy comforter from my back seat and fill my arms with the blue flannel. The blanket needs washing and I drag it down the hallway into the laundry room and slump down into it on the floor, in a puddle of me and flannel, my head pressing deep into the blue, cradling.

Then I remember I have wine in my room and decide I must drink it out of the bottle. I carry it through the house and sit outside in the hammock on the porch, staring up at the clouds that streak across the sky in slow motion.

I wish I liked alcohol. I wish I could drink the whole bottle of wine, get wasted, and have it all wash away. Instead, I get dizzy, put the wine down, drink some water, and soak in the Jacuzzi for a long time.

The birds populate the trees and tell their stories in a language I still don't understand. From the patio, I knock on Sebastian's window. My roommate keeps his door closed and plays video games all day. He declines my invitation to join me in the Jacuzzi.

Fine.

When Di gets off work, we cry on the phone together. We both felt alone today. I tell her that I think about suicide when my wheels spin along the highway. I think about smashing my car hard. I've found myself staring at my wrist while at a stoplight, the blue veins shining through like water. I'm not the suicide type, though. Obviously, I prefer a slow, torturous death.

*

I keep telling my dad that I'm an adult, and I can make it on my own.

He says, "You're acting like a fourteen-year-old."

I say, "Well, you're acting like a fourteen-year-old."

*

This atmosphere in this household is something new for me. Until now, other people have been the ones to initiate friendship with me.

Today, I decide I'll pursue Sebastian, not to date him but to be his friend, because I'm not happy, and I know he's not happy. Maybe we can find our own separate happiness being friends.

I want him to come with me to my secret spot, a cliff overhanging the ocean, to watch the stars. When I was younger, I would have gone there in the dark by myself and thought nothing of it, but now I realize the danger of being there alone at night. I decide to write him a note, and my heart beats wildly when my pen streaks the page, "Do you want to go to a cool place and watch the stars?" My feet pace back and forth in the hallway in front of his closed door, my heart pounding because the fear of rejection is so uncomfortable. I shove the note under his door and, like a fourteen-year-old, run back down the hallway.

I sit on the couch on the lanai, alternately journaling and watching the hallway. *Did he not see it?* I give up and go back to my room. A little later, his door opens and he walks down the hallway, out the front door, and gets in his car and drives away. *He completely ignored me.*

When he comes home with groceries a while later, I ignore him, which has no impact at all, since he's ignoring me. *Ouch. Screw it. I'll just leave him alone. That's what he wants anyway. Fine. I'll just send him love from afar.*

Now I have no one to go and watch the stars with me. *But God, I need to talk to the stars.*

Three nights later, Sebastian and I go and watch the stars. I first had to assure him that I had no romantic motives. I meant exactly what I'd written, "Hey, do you want to go watch the stars?" Literally.

We drive to the top of the cliff and sit down on the rocks with the sky spread out above and the sound of the ocean below. He gives me a little gift by sharing part of his story, which I hold delicately. We have a pretty hilarious laugh. It's the first time either of us has laughed in a while, and from that night on, we're friends.

69

WANDERERS

Tomorrow is Valentine's Day, and I return Leon's call during the ride home from my long day at work. He asks what my plans are for the weekend.

"I'm going to hang out with Di tonight. Then, I have that massage event tomorrow," I say, leaving out that I was planning on hanging out with Di tomorrow, too.

"Do you want to be my valentine?" he asks.

"Yes," I say, even though I'm thinking about Di. I do miss Leon's friendship. I fell in love with him because he made me happy when I wasn't happy. We were silly and fun. I do love him. I just can't feel it.

He says he misses me.

"Thanks. I miss you a little," I say. I want to say I miss him, but it would be a lie.

I'm a wanderer, a permanent traveler. It's what I do. It's what I like doing. It's full commitment temporarily. I enjoy the thrill of the constant flight, the happy memories. It's not that I don't believe in commitment—I do, but I also believe all of us should follow our own paths. I continue to wander and explore, because I'm still not sure exactly who I want to be.

Leon and I talk on the phone and agree to meet at the beach on Valentine's Day. We strain to find common ground for conversation over the next few minutes. When I hang up, I'm drained and wish I hadn't made plans with my mom for early the next morning.

*

My mom calls from the driveway when she arrives. I greet her outside and proceed to give her the tour of my new house. She's here for the first time to see where I live, and she walks around nodding, not saying much.

We drive to the marketplace for sushi and coffee as we make stupid conversation and tread water around the real issue.

Finally, I reach my limit. "You're not being honest with me, Mom. What do you want to say?"

"Dad didn't sleep all night, because he was up thinking of you two. And I was up crying."

"Why? It's not your life."

"It seems that you're spending all your time trying to fix your roommate's relationship when you don't even have a functioning one," she says.

What? I'm trying to be happy and peaceful. I'm enjoying the little things, such as buying what I want to eat for dinner, or my big bed, and my room where I can sing and play guitar, and the fact that I decorated it, and it's 100% mine.

*

My days consist of grudgingly getting up for work, leaving work as early as possible, racing home, and persuading a lazy Sebastian to accompany me to the lagoon. If the sun is still up and hot, we lie on the rocks like Komodo dragons and talk to each other with our eyes closed. Then, I jump off the log into the aqua blue water and find small shells on the sandy bottom of the bay. I bring them home as memory markers.

When I was little I'd swim at the neighborhood pool with my arms out like Superwoman and let my hair float wild underwater. All the little black tiles below me became rows of houses, and I would fly over them for as long as I could hold my breath.

Di and I call each other whenever we have breaks throughout the day. Usually, after work, I have some time to play guitar or read or relax until she calls, and we talk about our days while she rides around the mountain to my house, where we shower and I make dinner. The rest of the night is like a slumber party. We spend the time talking, laughing, crying, journaling, painting, watching movies, dancing in the kitchen, and trying to figure out our lives, until she goes home, a five minute drive away. We joke, "I'll call you in five minutes."

Many nights, my landlord has friends over, and we hang out with them, playing guitar or harmonizing songs and laughing and having conversations about God and the universe.

*

Tonight, on my way home from work, I stop by Leon's house to pick up some paperwork. As we talk, I want to collapse in puddles. I don't mean to be this person who shuts down when Leon talks to me. All I want to do is get my paperwork and leave, but I end up in the driveway with him ranting.

He takes off his ring and sets it on the concrete wall. He says he feels like he's the only one who is committed. He wants a reaction.

My expression doesn't waiver, even though I'm frantic inside. Instead, I shut down and judge myself for what a horrible person I am. I want everyone to stop pushing me.

He accuses me of not doing any work on myself and of being delusional.

Why do I say nothing? I'm hurting him. Why don't I feel anything? If I could, I'd scream. I'd force every last molecule of air from of my lungs and run. I want him to expect nothing. He loves me so much, but I've never had my freedom.

When we hug in the driveway, I'm full of tears on the inside but silent on the outside. Leon is crying.

Only when I'm alone in the car can I let myself break down and scream as I drive across the highway.

*

The light is on and all of my roommates' cars are at our house, so I take a few long breaths to compose myself before I enter. No one knows that I am fragile, uncertain, and on the verge of collapse.

Sebastian is making dinner in the kitchen, and I join him to talk for a while. Tonight, he's being mean to me, like a kid in second grade, joking but with a harsh undertone.

I poke him and say, "No swearing,"

He recoils, "Don't touch me."

"Stop being mean to me," I say.

He doesn't respond.

Uh, my heart hurts.

After a few minutes I make up some excuse to go to my room. The real reason is that I want to be wrapped up in a good friend's arms and cuddled in silence. I'm strong on the outside, but I'm hurting on the inside. Playing my guitar with the door closed doesn't help. Sitting in the dark in the shower crying doesn't work. *God, I'm vulnerable. I want a hug from someone I trust, who will treat me like the fragile little girl I feel I am right now and protect me and keep me safe and happy.*

In my dreams I run with all that's left in me, down the jagged swooping rocks, before I reach the cliff. And this time I don't stop. I jump, arms out, following through without hesitation, wholeheartedly taking the plunge into the ocean.

I shouldn't have married Leon. I'm not making it complicated. It is complicated. If he understood what I'm fighting for, then he wouldn't ask me to mold myself into someone else.

Like a harpoon shot through water, I awake gasping, in the middle of my huge bed, the candle flames dancing against the window.

70

THE SEEDS ARE SO PRETTY

Faith. Trust. Love.
I have the seeds.
The seeds, they are so pretty.
Why can't I find good dirt?
Who will love me?
Who will water me?
(Di)

"Dad said he thinks you hate him. He said that you want him out of your life."

My mom and I are eating shave ice.

"Um. First of all, that's not true, and second, that doesn't sound like something I would say."

"Maybe you should call him," she says.

So I call him to clear up these misunderstandings. He gives me one-word answers to "How's your day going?" and my other questions, and then he goes silent.

"Do you not want to talk to me?" I say.

"I have nothing to say to you anymore. You're a different person. I don't even know you anymore."

"Well, why don't you try to get to know the new me?"

"I have no interest in getting to know people like you. You are completely different." He imagines that he's failed as a parent because he can't instruct me. "We used to be so connected," he says, "and now we aren't at all."

I'm proud of myself, because I take his criticism in, open-mouthed, and manage to respond, "OK, well, if you want to connect to me, I'm here. If you decide you want to get to know the new me."

I hang up confused. *And he wonders why I don't call him.*

Why does my dad act insulted, as though he's failed as a parent? He doesn't want to get to know me without my eating disorder. My parents liked the seed of me, but now they don't like the tree that I've grown into.

It's OK. God made me. God will water me.

I focus on having a great day with my mom. It starts off great with the two of us laughing about home movies and sharing shave ice and walking home in the sun and the breeze. My mom gives me an at-home pedicure as we watch old videos of us camping at Waimānalo beach when I was a little kid.

Leon calls to ask about my plan for summer, because he's debating whether or not to take an internship in California. I don't know my plan.

When I get off the phone, my mom's energy has shifted, and she's no longer in the mood to be my friend. She has become the parent. "It seems like everything is about Di now," she says. "What about Leon?"

I don't want to answer. *We were having such a great day.*

My mom waits for an answer.

I focus on the thick paper she has laid out for me, and the paint she has provided, hoping she'll drop the subject, but I feel my anger building. When I snap, I become a feral child. My words escape aggressively though gritted teeth.

She won't stop talking.

On the table in front of me is a blank, pure white canvas. My eyes focus on it to muffle the background noise. My hands place puddles of color on a plate, different happy colors in dime-like circles. Nothing comes. Nothing comes. My mind blurs. I shut down.

Leon asked me angrily the other night, "When have you ever been alone?"

But alone is when you can't share yourself with others.

Watching those old videos, I'd thought, *Maybe I was never a normal kid.* In them, my brother was talking, laughing, bouncing while I looked away from the camera. In some shots, I appeared aloof and bossy, as if I had all the confidence in the world and I didn't care. I looked like a child actor switching expressions on cue.

The blank white paper makes me think of a blizzard. The snow absorbs my screams. I begin putting my paintbrush on the page, hoping my subconscious will connect the dots. Even though I want to crumple it up and begin again, I keep going.

From the unintentional life that I started with, I will make something.

In one of Robert Frost's poems[2], "the best way out is always through."

So, I add more color. Shapes begin to form hidden letters. When I connect the dots, they spell, "Help me." I can see the words clearly, even though I conceal them with light and shadow, as though the sky is burning down like a bad acid trip. I am the figure on the rock. I have purple skin and my trademark multicolored hair. I have a signature representation of myself in art. I'm a figure, always facing away from the viewer. Most of my body is draped with my long rainbow-colored hair.

*

Later that night, when Di looks at my picture, she nods, "Yeah. It's like you're saying, 'You never know what's inside me unless I tell you how to look at me.'"

---

[2] Frost, Robert. "A Servant to Servants" in *North of Boston* (New York: Henry Holt, 1917), p. 64.

71

CHOICE

"If you believe, you will get anything you ask for in prayer."
Matthew 21:22 GNT

In recovery, the only thing that stopped me from throwing up was seeing the future I wanted—that dinner in Italy with my friends, smiling, laughing, being truly happy. It was the moment that I had to visualize when I was too full and the eating disorder was triggered. I had to tell myself, *Just this once. Keep it down this once, and that will be your life*. Each time I succeeded, I felt closer to the future I pictured in my head, one choice at a time.

For the last two weeks, Leon and I have been giving each other space. The funny thing is that when he stopped trying to get me back, suddenly I began thinking about him again.

I've been observing my roommate with a critical eye and cultivating a lot of respect and admiration for the amazing person Leon is—loving and playful and willing to go with the flow. I'm appreciating him and his love, sacrifice, and motivation. He's smart, mature, ethical. He loves God, and he's silly and goofy and fun.

I've been looking for someone just like me, perhaps a male mirror of me. I've wanted someone to be able to connect to every single part of me, but I'm coming to see that it's not possible. We have different friends, because no one person can fill us completely. Expecting one person to be everything is handing the responsibility for my happiness to someone else. It's dangerous. Instead, I can hold my happiness like pebbles in my hands, and I can extend my hands to someone and say, "Hey, here's my stuff. I'd like to show it to you. I'd like to invite you to take a look at it." I'm realizing how important it is to hold my own sense of self-worth and happiness and not surrender it to anyone else.

I've read somewhere that the amount of abuse you'll tolerate from others is just a little less than the amount you abuse yourself. I used to abuse myself a lot. Now I'm nicer to myself.

I haven't thrown up in months. At first, I was too scared to clog the toilets and have my new housemates find out I have an eating disorder, but there's another part of me that is stronger, that wants to get and stay better, that wants the promise of a new life. I know that if I can rid myself of Lillie, happiness is attainable.

I give other people way too much credit. In the end, they do what they want to do.

Liza says that my responsibility is to be honest about my boundaries, put them out there as kindly and responsibly as possible, and then trust that most people can tolerate my honesty. I'll learn quickly who is safe and who is not.

When I tell her about my parents, she reassures me that all eating disorder patients go through this phase of learning how to set healthy boundaries. Most of our lives have been lived in black and white extremes, and we don't know how to live in the middle.

*

I sometimes worry that I'm being rude when I shut my bedroom door. I'm concerned that my housemates will feel shut out. *This is crazy. I can't believe I'm debating the significance of shutting my bedroom door.* My bedroom door has become a perfect symbol of my desire for both openness and privacy.

72

MANIFEST

"You're much less angry than you used to be," Liza tells me in today's therapy session.

"Thank you?" I wonder how angry I used to seem, if I'm less angry now.

The past week, especially, people have been commenting on my ass, and I want to say, *Fuck you,* but instead I say, "Thank you," roll my eyes, and turn away.

My pants grip around my ass and thighs. *Too big, too big.*

Lillie shakes her head. "Your ass is too large. You're a failure, a disappointment. You can't do anything right."

No. OK, so my ass is larger than I'd like. So what. My happiness comes from within my spirit.

"Failure."

It takes all my therapy, my whole bag of tools, to fight all day long against Lillie's voice in my head. She's so cruel. I'm exhausted by the time I get home. It feels like, instead of having gone to work, I spent the past seven hours not giving in to torture.

I cry and cry, but I do not throw up. I do not throw up.

*

After talking to Leon this week, I drive home to music that makes me want to burst into water and dissolve through the cracks in the leather seats. I try to avoid his calls, but it's easier to answer the phone than to take the flak later for ignoring him.

Conversations with Leon on my long drive home make me feel like I'm drowning. I tell him I want to end the conversation, but he pushes for an answer. "What do you think about this? What do you feel? What do you have to say?" In the flood, everything is underwater. My thoughts slosh back and forth incoherently. Like trying to read someone's lips in a swimming pool, I see the bubbles but I can't make out the words.

I don't know how I feel. Just let me get off the damn phone.

When I get the OK, finally, I slam the off button and throw my phone on the floorboard, not caring that the face pops off.

I don't look my housemate in the eyes as I ascend the stairs with my hair in my face, so he can't see that I've been crying. I fix my voice long enough to make it down the hallway to the haven of my room. Door closed and locked, I turn on the song "Bizarre Love Triangle," which reminds me of my childhood, and listen to it over and over and over and over and over and over. My blue pillowcase is darkened with tears. I fall asleep clutching my pink crystal that symbolizes love.

73

I LOVE TREES

The more Leon and I try to work towards getting back together, the more I realize we don't connect on much of anything anymore. I'd like to share with him that I found a shaman lady who teaches classes. I'd like to share things about my conversations with Di and my roommate Sebastian. But either my effort goes nowhere or I have to guard what I say. When I talk, he has a habit of not responding. Still, we try.

It's mostly his idea, but we have one dinner a week together as a quasi date night, to keep the communication open, to keep hanging by a thread onto the fragile hope of reconciliation. Indian food is tonight's cuisine that we bring to the park and eat under the pretty trees with mushroom tops.

"I like trees," Leon says. "They remind me of wisdom."

"I love trees," I say. "I think I was a tree."

No response.

We go back to his house to look at condos for a vacation my parents gave us as a present. As if a few days away together could fix this. I've brought my stuff to sleep over, but he says something about wanting to go to bed early.

Stupid girl. Why did you just assume you were going to stay? Stupid, stupid, stupid.

Without thinking, because I want to share with Leon, I pull up on the computer some pictures of my friend's bachelorette party, forgetting the one picture of me being given a fifteen-second piggyback ride by one of the guys that bought our group drinks. It was a joke. It was funny. That's all it was.

But Leon gets upset. "You're a bad wife," he says. "That's totally unacceptable. That's flirting with another guy."

"It was a joke," I say. *What the fuck? It was nothing.*

We don't talk after that, because I disagree and there's no way to win. I sit on the couch as he's fiddling in the closet with the door open. I realize he's loading his pockets with his keys and his wallet.

"I'm going to get ice cream," he says.

Does that mean me, too? I like ice cream.

"Can you lock up on the way out," he says, because I still have a key.

"Yes." *Try to pretend it doesn't bother you.*

Lillie smiles, "Stupid, fat, worthless fake. Liar. Disappointment. Failure. No one wants you, stupid little girl."

I wait barely long enough for him to exit the driveway before I walk out, lock the door, and drive home.

I don't know what to do about our situation. Why can't we just be happy? Why is it that I connect more with a random stranger in fifty minutes at the spa today than I do with my husband of six years?

Who am I?

I am my soul that loves me. God is proud of me and holds me close under His protective wings.

*

Even though things look bleak, Leon and I agree to take a trip together. As an early anniversary present, my parents have rented us a vacation condo for the weekend. The two of us watch movies, relax, eat, and lie by the pool. We go through the motions, doing the things that made us feel connected in the past. In the present, it feels like somehow I ended up at the pool with a stranger. There are long stretches of silence. I read a book about numerology, and he swims.

But in the silence, I begin to observe him and think about us. Then, like magic, a few things become clear.

Is it possible that I'm projecting problems on Leon that are my responsibility to fix?

Like, number one, the fact that I associate Leon with my eating disorder, so I find myself reverting back to my old mindset and emotional state when I'm with him.

Like, number two, the fact that Leon doesn't have to flow with me all the time, agree with me, or even discuss certain things with me. By putting so much emphasis on these things, I'm doing exactly what I hate when he does it to me. I'm expecting him to be someone he's not. Then, I get disappointed when he's not who I want him to be. There can be no double standards here. If I choose to love him, I choose to love him fully for exactly who he is.

Like, number three, the fact that I've placed too much significance on this trip, as though it's my deciding factor as to whether we have a future together.

In church, I once learned that the Israelites were just an eleven-day journey from reaching the promised land, but they wandered around the same mountain for thirty-seven years, because God wanted the people to rely on Him and not to think about returning to Egypt during difficult or frightening times.

How many times have I circled the same mountain, when I was so close to where I was supposed to be?

When I prayed to God, I wasn't magically healed. I had to crawl around the mountain of my eating disorder for eleven years. It took time to work the anger out of my heart. It took time to be open and able to receive what God had for me all along. His plan was bigger than magically healing me overnight. If He had, I wouldn't have appreciated it.

*

Di's uncle said something powerful to me the other day. He said that the old-school way of dealing with marriage conflict was to resolve miscommunication. The old method doesn't work for us, because Leon and I actually communicate well. The problem is that we are entirely different people with incompatible goals. Her uncle said that the new way of dealing with marriage conflict is to find the positive. "It's about the positive qualities outweighing the negative. It's about having a storehouse of positive experiences and memories made together that bond a couple."

While we were in California, our marriage was horrible for both of us, and a lot of that trauma has shrouded the happiness we once shared.

I was an addict. I was never fully present. Lillie was talking to me all day, like white noise. That's why my memories are fuzzy. They're overshadowed by my addiction.

Leon and I, together, need to create new, positive, happy memories with new experiences, conversations, and laughter. *We need to build a new storehouse.*

In the condo, after midnight, in the white sheets that remind me of clouds, I stare at the ceiling. Love is the sum of our choices, and we can always make different ones at any point in time. I've done a lot of damage, but Leon still loves me. Because of that, I know it's not too late. I choose to refill our storehouse of happiness one grain at a time, even if I have to scale the walls to throw them in. I want Leon to be with the real me, because she's here now. I've worked hard to find her. He's loved all of me, even when it hurt him. He should be around to reap the benefits of my growth.

When I stare at the ceiling, I think about love and the new things that grow after a heavy rain.

74

OPEN MY HEART

In the condo, after midnight, in the white sheets that remind me of clouds, Leon shifts in his sleep. He hugs his white pillow as a cute little moan escapes his lips, and he reaches across the sky filled with clouds, over the fluffy white oceans of waves. He reaches for my hand to hold it.

Even after all I've put him through, he still loves me. In the dark, half asleep, he reaches for my hand, wanting to be close to me.

My heart implodes with the magnitude of love, knowing that people love you and stay with you even when you think you're horrible and ugly inside, even when you're at your worst.

I feel the warmth of his hand. *This person has loved me and stayed.* I want to be here with him now, and I want to stay. He deserves the best of me.

*

Before Leon and I make the decision to move back in together, I ask God for insight. Should I study with the shaman lady I found during the quest for wise women to follow?

That night, He gives me a dream. In the dream, I sit cross-legged in front of the shaman. Everything is fine until I go against her wishes; then, she has the power to hurt me.

In my dream, I ask the shaman a question. She leans towards me and places her index fingers in my ears. My left ear feels normal, but on the right

I notice something strange—a claw.

Immediately I jolt awake, as the candle flames dizzily dance in the dimness, a clock chimes, and shadows sway. I know the answer.

Over the next few days, I give away most of the books on my bookshelf, because they've been leaning steadily towards the occult. I throw away all my crystals. I rebuke all dark energies, and everything changes.

One week after my dream, Leon and I are talking about when I'm going to move back.

As I pack my things, I'm grateful for my time spent wandering in search of answers, because what I found connected me to the love of God without guilt. God is the thread that I held onto, that held me together, that kept me sane. He's the one who makes all things good, who takes the broken pieces and glues them back together to make something new and beautiful.

For over eleven years I abused my body and my mind and yet they still function. I owe this, absolutely, to God watching over me and protecting me from all the harm I did to myself. He has kept me safe, so I can share my story, so other people will know that true freedom is possible. God is present. He is awesome love.

"If you are going through hell," Winston Churchill said, "keep going." My friend Mel told me repeatedly, "You have to go through the hate to get to the love." Now, I understand that there are no shortcuts. There is no way out but through.

I look at the words in blue marker that I wrote three months ago on the mirror. I copied them from my college journal, so I wouldn't forget God's promise. Now, many years later, it's finally coming true:

I have a gift for you but you must be patient
Quiet your soul.
I am with you always.
I love you.

75

THE BEGINNING

"A glass of Twisted, please," I say, choosing from the selection of specialty wines for the morbid curiosity one label invokes. We're celebrating our seventh anniversary dinner with a night out at a cozy Italian restaurant. I stop laughing long enough to take a drink. It slides down my throat: dry, medium tannins. I'm grateful for the spaces that are now full. A glass of wine, insalata Caprese, grilled vegetable panini with Havarti cheese and pesto mayonnaise, mesclun greens, flourless chocolate addiction cake, my husband's face—a smile spreads like water across my lips as I think of the distance I've traversed.

I hear myself in the distance, *Hi, my name is Christen, and I am finally free.*

I see the faces of the women sitting around the hospital tables, wearing their smiles like tattoos of honor, as they shout in unison, "Yes, you are!"

EPILOGUE

Thank you. Thank you. Thank you, God. My heart is overflowing with joy.

"Where's my popcorn?" Leon says for the third time with a smile in his voice.

"I will punch you in the face." I laugh as I turn on the stove.

We sit side by side in our chairs, eating popcorn and watching TV. It's a simple moment but it's monumental. One different choice and this moment would not exist; we would not be here, continuing our life together. This is joy. The little seeds that have taken root in my heart and grown into this tree we share, our life. Even though we may not have it all together all the time, God has blessed us. Together, we have it all.

"What?" he says looking over.

"Nothing. I just love you."

"Why?"

"Because you're so cute."

"Thanks," he says, reaching forward like a sloth to pick up a big handful of popcorn. He glances at me sideways and rapidly shoves it into his mouth, pretending I didn't see.

"That's my line." I say.

"I love you, too," he says.

"Thanks," I say, with a huge smile.

*

In the Bible, Paul talks about how each man's work will be tested by fire, and if what he has built survives, he will receive his reward.

I watch the house that Lillie and I built burn to the ground. She tries to talk to me but her voice dissipates in the smoke. The flames engulf it all, and I walk away, past the onlookers, down the block to where it is quiet and dark except for the streetlights overhead.

"So, do you know where you're going, or are you just blindly going out in the dark?"

I look up to see a raven perched on a streetlamp. I smile and exhale. This time, I know exactly where I'm going—home.

This is my choice. Leon and me.

THOUGHTS ON MARRIAGE

Marriage, like recovery, is a choice. When we choose to do everything we can to cultivate and then stay long enough to see the seeds grow, happiness can be present instead of unattainably distant. Staying is the hard part because it feels like a war. But after war is peace.

ACKNOWLEDGEMENTS: MAHALO AND ALOHA

Writing my memoir has been a fortunate journey of insight. Through the process I was able to look back at my own immaturity and laugh and cry at what showed up on the pages. Mahalo to all those who have generously allowed me to share pieces of their truths.

Incredibly deep thanks to the women and men who worked at the hospital where I was treated. I'm filled with awe and admiration of your support when we're at our worst. My time with you instilled the bright spark of hope.

To the amazing friends I made in the hospital, I adore you. Thanks for cracking me up with your dark and witty charm, for lessons learned through our tears, for sharing your hearts and stories, for accepting me with love, and for telling me that I was strong. I still smile when I recall our freedom ceremony and our '80s wristbands. You were the first people I'd ever been honest with about my deepest secret, and I'm so glad it was you. "No more secrets. No more pain. Live on!"

Thank you to the handful of caring therapists I've had over the course of my recovery. The difference you make is akin to throwing a starfish back into the ocean so it can live.

Liza Wacker, the wonderful therapist whose couch became my home for a year, you sat patiently as I ranted but could silence me with a single word. Thanks for teaching me to ride the waves. I always pictured you smiling at the memo I wrote on my checks: "to fix my brain." My gratitude is immense. It fills my heart and spans the worlds of my mind.

To the spa community, thank you for providing the best playground to explore and grow in a safe and loving environment. All the experiences and conversations brought me clarity on what I wanted for my life and gave me insight into the person I longed to be. Without realizing it, you supported me through one of the most difficult times in my life. I deeply appreciate you all. *Mahalo nui loa.*

To Leon's dad, grandma, and sister. You showed me love at its best. I was stunned by your acceptance, despite my behavior during our imploding relationship, and will never forget how odd and wonderful it felt. Love you guys.

To the man with the Golden Ticket, who opened my eyes, proved magic was possible, and granted me an adventure. Thank you. I remember my part.

To Ani DiFranco, whose luminous words and emphatic guitar buoyed my deflated heart.

To the friends who rock my world with laughter, honesty, and open hearts. Julie, soon we will have been friends for longer than we haven't been. There's certain magic in being present through various incarnations of ourselves. Mel, pretty *wahine,* in all our adventures and travels you never cease to wow me with your strength, vulnerability, and willingness to stay present and do the work. Your objective insight was invaluable and delivered with the softest care. Di, feather, you have taught me to live from my heart instead of my brain. Here's to treehouses in the forest, a villa in Italy, and watching the valley burn. I love you, period.

To my family, who gifted me with a most gorgeous childhood, I cherish your constant support, laughing at the darkness, and showing me the light. Thanks for encouraging me to write the truth and season it with love. You are where my happiest memories reside. I love you tons—more than dirt.

To Leon, who's shown me the blessing and power of being steadfast, when I say that you ground me, I mean that you are the roots that nourish me. Of all the many paths my life might have taken, I'm elated this one brought me home to you.

To my previous agent, Robin M., who lit the fire under me and encouraged me to build stamina for a marathon, not a sprint, thank you for your insight, for believing in this story, for being present for every step, and for telling me the truth, with love.

To Robin C., my editor, who laughed with me as we reworked the pages.

To Lisa Chaly for the cover photo and many fabulous photo shoots.

To Marisa Bean for creative logo design.

To the friends who do not appear on the pages of this book, you are present, nonetheless, between the lines. You fill my life with belly laughs, wisdom, escapades, and joy. May we have an abundance of them all.

To God, awesome and everywhere and always orchestrating a beautiful harmony from the cacophonous chaos of me, You didn't heal me magically like I'd always wanted, but Your plan was better because I learned.

To Lillie, my eating disorder, without whom this book couldn't have been written, I appreciate all you taught me, and I'm not sorry to have bid you goodbye.

For those on the outside looking in, may you find insight and compassion while supporting those you love. Thank you for being here and caring.

For those still struggling with an eating disorder, you are the reason this book exists. You are far braver than you know. Even though we've never met, I love you. I wish you freedom.

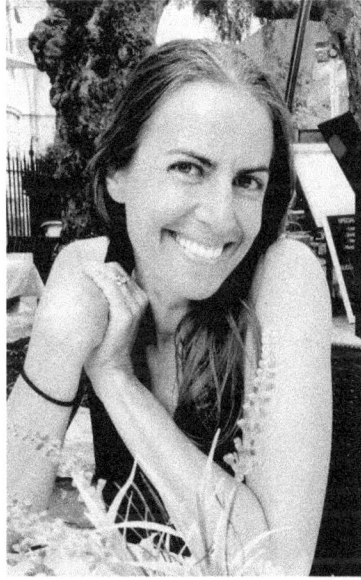

Z Zoccolante loves belly laughs, starry skies, chocolate chip cookies, and is deeply fascinated by a well-written fairytale villain. Originally from Hawai'i, she lives in LA pursuing her multi-faceted dreams and training as a therapist specializing in addiction recovery. In her free time, you can find her reading books in her bikini and adventuring with her dog. Her podcast Throwing Up Rainbows on iTunes, reveals the secret world of eating disorders told through her personal stories.

Visit her at zzoccolante.com.

www.ingramcontent.com/pod-product-compliance
Lightning Source LLC
Chambersburg PA
CBHW020248030426
42336CB00010B/677